Eugenia S. Medina

C000080173

PRACTICAL GENERAL MEDICINE

With the compliments of Rorer Pharmaceuticals Ltd.

Tex. 94

PRACTICAL GENERAL MEDICINE

CARDIOVASCULAR AND RESPIRATORY DISEASES
QUESTIONS AND ANSWERS

BY

D.G. MODEL
BSc FRCP

Consultant Physician
Eastbourne Health Authority

Cole and Whurr
London and New Jersey

Copyright © 1989
Cole and Whurr Limited
19b Compton Terrace
London N1 2UN
England

First published 1989

All rights reserved. This book is protected by
copyright. No part of this book may be
reproduced in any form or by any means,
including photocopying, or utilised by any
information storage or retrieval system without
written permission from the copyright owner.

British Library Cataloguing in Publication Data

Model, D.G.
    Pratical general medicine
    1. Man. Cardiovascular system. Diseases
    2. Man. Respiratory system. Diseases
    I. Title
    616.1

    ISBN 1-871381-14-2

Typeset by Maggie Spooner Typesetting, London
Printed in Great Britain by Mackays of Chatham

Contents

Acknowledgements

I should like to thank Dr Paul Curry of Guy's Hospital and Dr Alistair Macleod of Eastbourne for many helpful comments about the cardiovascular section of the book, and Dr John Collins of the Brompton Hospital for valued advice about the respiratory section. Special thanks are also due to Dr Sayar Molki for the illustrations, and to Mrs Ann Manners, Mrs Margaret Kinnear and Mrs Heather Higgins for so patiently typing the text.

This book is dedicated to the students from all over the world whom it has been my privilege to teach, and to my wife for allowing me to hide away at weekends to write it.

Introduction

In ordinary clinical practice patients present, doctors take histories and examine them, and hopefully only when indicated, order investigations. From these encounters questions arise. At an everyday level these are likely to be about the diagnosis, what investigations, if any, should be ordered, and what treatment if any might be appropriate? All this is against the background of a broad spectrum of possible underlying pathologies. This book reflects these everyday processes. To achieve this a format has been adopted in which cases are presented, questions are asked and answers are provided.

Apart from reflecting the everyday diagnostic process the book also aims to increase students' contribution to their learning. Being a student is not easy for a young adult. At a time when their peers with ordinary jobs are already contributing to society through their work, the student is still on the receiving end, contributing very little except for the requirement to keep passively absorbing knowledge like a sponge. In a sense of course, learning from a textbook is an active process, although it is one that many students find difficult and dull despite a wish to learn. This book aims to help overcome this problem. By asking for answers to specific questions it is hoped to focus the student's attention and stimulate him or her to contribute more actively and more specifically to the process of learning.

Based as it is upon case histories, the book is not intended to cover every aspect of cardiovascular and respiratory disease, but rather to look at a large number of common medical conditions in depth. The questions asked have been carefully designed and are of a very different type to the questions asked in most books of multiple choice. In the latter the questions are usually haphazard and often deal with minutiae which makes integrated learning difficult. In the present book the questions have been arranged to lead on from one to another in such a way that the answers cover the whole of each subject and can be read in much the same way as a standard textbook.

A special effort has been made to present the data in a readily accessible visual form that hopefully will reduce the student's need to underline the text.

Technical subjects are most easily learned by thinking in terms of pictures. In this book a special effort has been made to facilitate picture thinking by presenting concepts in terms of pictures and word images, and by presenting the underlying physiology and tissue pathology of the conditions dealt with. However, being an effective clinician also involves having a large mass of often disparate facts at one's finger tips. For most people the best way of learning these facts is by repeatedly reading them and forming them into lists. For this reason no apology is made for asking questions that oblige students to list their answers, or for presenting parts of the text in the form of lists.

Lists have their limitations, but learning involves both acquiring knowledge and getting it into disciplined order, and lists help this process. In a way they are also germinal to the diagnostic process, which is largely a matter of recognising patterns of symptoms, signs and investigations. The division into specific diseases with names of the vast spectrum of symptoms and signs with which we are presented is largely a mental convenience that enables us to organise our thoughts and recognise particular groups or patterns of symptoms, signs and investigations that we have been taught or have learned to label as particular conditions. The best diagnosticians are those who are thorough and have an innate gift together with a large mass of understood ordered facts from which to pick the patterns.

Perhaps this seems dull. It isn't. Fortunately for our interest as doctors, though not always for the good of our patients, the interactions between the diverse ways illness presents and the people it affects are so varied that the patterns it throws up are a never ending source of interest and stimulation.

Case A

A Case of Breathlessness: Mrs A-B, aged 62 years

A widow living alone in a neat ground floor apartment built halfway up a moderately steep hill with a parade of local shops at the bottom.

History of present condition

Referred by her family practitioner for assessment of breathlessness for which he could not find a cause. The patient herself complained of several attacks of what she called 'bronchitis' during the preceding winter. By this she meant episodes, lasting several days, of breathlessness on exertion without the production of sputum.

More recently she had been breathless every time she walked up the slope to her home from the local shops, and on one or two occasions had woken at about 1 a.m. with a dry cough and slight breathlessness. During the previous day or so she had noticed that she was breathless about her home and even when talking. She had also noticed that during the previous two weeks her feet and ankles had become increasingly swollen, and that she had continuous slight discomfort in her upper abdomen unrelated to eating or opening her bowels.

Past medical history

Fourteen years previously she had been found to be hypertensive when she was being assessed for iritis that subsequently resolved spontaneously.

Relevant direct questions

Chest pain: nil.
Smoking: seven cigarettes per day.
Micturition: nocturia × 1 or 2 for about 6 months (negative for sugar).
Drugs: A proprietary drug for her hypertension, containing 100 mg of the beta blocking drug, atenolol, and 5 mg of the diuretic, hydrochlorothiazide.

Examination

Well looking middle-aged lady who nonetheless was short of breath when moving about the room. On general examination there was no obvious cyanosis but there was oedema up to the thighs.

Cardiovascular system (CVS)

The main clinical findings were:
Pulse 80 regular, good volume.
Blood pressure (BP) 140/90 lying and standing.
Jugular venous pulse (JVP) 6 cm above the manubrio/sternal angle
with the patient lying back at an angle of approximately 45
degrees.

On palpation

Apex: sustained and displaced to the anterior axillary line in the
sixth intercostal space.
Right ventricle: an abnormal heave.

On auscultation

The only abnormality was a gallop third heart sound heard just
medially to the apex.

Respiratory system (RS)

At the lung bases a few late inspiratory crackles were audible.

Mrs A-B
Questions

1   What was the diagnosis in Mrs A-B's case?
2i   What do you think was the cause of the discomfort in the
upper part of her abdomen?
ii   What was the likeliest cause of Mrs A-B's nocturia? How
may it be explained?
3   Comment on a possible connection between the patient's
condition and the drugs she was taking.

Answers

1   The diagnosis of Mrs A-B's case

The history of breathlessness and swelling of the ankles, associated
with a raised jugular venous pulse, marked cardiomegaly and late
inspiratory crackles at the lung bases all indicate that Mrs A-B was
suffering from congestive cardiac failure, a term that is usually used
to mean both left and right heart failure.

However, a diagnosis such as *congestive cardiac failure* or *left
ventricular failure* is not complete as it does not imply an
underlying cause for the condition. Because so many underlying
causes of heart failure are reversible it is important to try to
identify the cause of the condition. In Mrs A-B's case this was
almost certainly hypertension.

Comments on the history and physical findings

●   Taking a history involves an act of great imagination, of
imagining oneself to be the patient, sharing his or her experience,

and asking about the time of day, where the patient was, and what they were doing when the complaint began.

It also involves never accepting the use of words by the patient such as 'angina', 'bronchitis', 'indigestion', 'asthma', or 'migraine', without clearly establishing what is meant, because, for instance, to many patients 'migraine' is any severe headache, 'angina' may mean breathlessness, and 'indigestion' may cover a spectrum of symptoms from burping to severe pain. In the present instance Mrs A-B used the word 'bronchitis' to mean breathlessness on exertion without the production of any sputum. Her own family doctor accepted this uncritically, whereas most physicians would associate the term 'bronchitis' with the production of sputum. Most probably, of course, her breathlessness during the previous winter was due to episodes of pulmonary congestion resulting from left ventricular failure.

● Presumably the family doctor had not examined her. Had he done so he would no doubt easily have made the correct diagnosis.

2i   The discomfort in the upper part of Mrs A-B's abdomen

This was almost certainly due to right heart failure causing congestion of the liver and stretching and stimulation of the rich nerve supply to its capsule.

2ii   Mrs A-B's nocturia

Nocturia may be due to many conditions including cardiac failure which was most probably the cause in Mrs A-B's case. The explanation of this is that oedematous states such as cardiac failure and the nephrotic syndrome are associated with the retention of salt and water, some of which leaves dependent areas such as the legs when the patient lies flat and enters the vascular compartment where it acts like a saline infusion and is excreted by the kidneys. Indeed, in some patients with oedema due to hypoproteinaemia it has been shown that lying supine with the legs elevated has a therapeutically useful diuretic effect, that is even greater in patients who lie supine in a tilting position with the head down.

3   A possible connection between Mrs A-B's condition and the drugs she was taking

Although the underlying cause of Mrs A-B's heart failure was hypertension the beta blocking drug she was taking also probably contributed to her condition through its negative inotropic action. Full details of the actions and side effects of these drugs are given on page 100.

Chapter 1
Symptoms and Signs in Cardiac Disease

Questioning the patient; an explanation of oedema
Questions

1   Apart from using one's imagination when taking a history, and trying to share the patient's experience, making a correct diagnosis is often facilitated by knowing what specific direct questions to ask about the disease or system suspected of malfunction. In the present instance list the *specific* direct questions that should be asked in a case of suspected cardiac disease. Give your reasons for asking them.

2   Explain the mechanism in the capillaries by which oedema fluid collects in the legs in cardiac failure.

Answers

1   The direct questions that should be asked in a case of suspected cardiac disease

These questions are designed to aid diagnosis and help in assessing the severity of the condition. Always ask specifically about:

●   *Chest pain?* Angina of effort, myocardial infarction and acute pericardial disease are typified by chest pain. A full discussion of the differential diagnosis of chest pain is given on page 82.

●   *Breathlessness on exertion or at rest?* There are many causes of breathlessness and a full discussion of their differential diagnosis is given on page 217. From a cardiological point of view, breathlessness is a common symptom of pulmonary congestion due to left ventricular failure. The mechanism of this and the various patterns of breathlessness associated with left ventricular failure are discussed on page 9 in the answer to question 4.

●   *Nocturnal breathlessness?* Because patients often omit to mention this, it is important to ask specifically about nocturnal dyspnoea which may be a symptom of cardiac failure, although more commonly it is a symptom of bronchial asthma.

●   *Swelling of the ankles?* As explained on page 32, cardiac failure is associated with the retention of salt and water, most of which accumulate behind the ventricle that has failed. In right heart failure this leads to an accumulation of fluid in the systemic veins which as described in the next answer results in peripheral oedema.

●   *Palpitations?* Interpretation of this symptom is difficult because many people with a normal heart rhythm are aware of their heart beat, especially in bed with their head on the pillow.

Nonetheless, a history of palpitations should arouse suspicion of an arrhythmia. An indication of the speed and rhythm of the palpitation may be obtained by getting the patient to tap out what they feel on their chest or on a table. A full discussion of arrhythmias is given on page 54.

● *Dizziness or unconsciousness?* These symptoms may be of either circulatory or neurological cause. Dizziness and syncope of circulatory cause are due to decreased perfusion of the brain. The commonest circulatory causes of dizziness or syncope are:

a   Vasovagal attack (fainting).
b   Postural hypotension due to drugs or, more rarely, autonomic neuropathy.
c   Tachyarrhythmia.
d   Heart block.
e   Valvular stenosis—particularly aortic stenosis.

2   Mechanism within the capillaries leading to the formation of oedema

In right heart failure the accumulation of fluid within the systemic veins causes the hydrostatic pressure at the venous end of the capillaries to rise above the oncotic pressure exerted by the plasma proteins. As a consequence fluid is not drawn back into the vasculature at the venous end of the capillaries but instead collects in the interstitial spaces where under the influence of gravity it drains to the legs.

Breathlessness and the abnormal patterns of breathing associated with cardiac failure

Questions

3i   Breathlessness is a common symptom of cardiac disease. Define the term 'breathlessness'. How is the sensation we know as breathlessness perceived by the nervous system?
ii   List the chemical and neurological stimuli of *ventilation*. At what sites in the nervous system do they act?
4i   What are the main mechanisms causing the breathlessness associated with left ventricular failure?
ii   List the various abnormal patterns of breathing seen in patients with left ventricular failure, and explain the additional mechanisms (over and above those mentioned in the first part of your answer) that contribute to them.
5   Describe Cheyne-Stokes repiration. How may it be explained physiologically? In what conditions is it encountered?

Answers

3i   Breathlessness

This is defined as an abnormal and uncomfortable awareness of breathing. Although as indicated in the answer to the second part of this question a great deal is known about the various stimuli of ventilation, little is known about the mechanisms producing the sensation we know as breathlessness. Perhaps the most attractive hypothesis is that breathlessness is a sensation produced when the demand on the lungs is greater than their capacity to respond, or when the tension developed by the respiratory muscles is excessive in relation to their movement. But how this is signalled to the cerebral cortex and on which area of the cortex it is perceived is not known.

3ii Stimulation of ventilation

By comparison with other striated muscles, to an unparalleled extent the anterior horn cells of the respiratory muscles are served by two upper motor neurones—one from the respiratory centre in the medulla, the other from the cerebral cortex. With this in mind the stimuli of ventilation may be summarised as follows and as illustrated in Figure 1.

● *Carbon dioxide and hydrogen ions* acting directly to stimulate the respiratory centre.

● *Anoxia* acting indirectly via fibres that run in the glossopharyngeal or IXth cranial nerve to the respiratory centre from specialised oxygen sensing cells in the carotid body and to a lesser extent the aortic body.

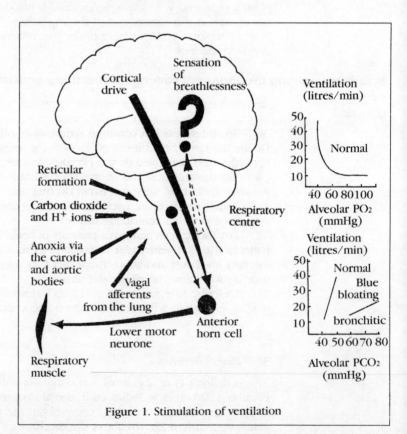

Figure 1. Stimulation of ventilation

- *Sensory fibres* that run from the lung to the respiratory centre in branches of the vagus or Xth cranial nerve, and indirectly stimulate the respiratory centre with impulses from irritant and stretch receptors in the lung and receptors that sense engorgement of the pulmonary capillaries.
- *The reticular formation* conveying information about the state of arousal of the individual. It is this pathway that is associated with the increased ventilation that occurs when we are awake.
- *Cortical drive* allowing an element of conscious control of ventilation, and ventilation to vary with fear, pain, breath holding and activities such as speech and the performance of lung function tests.

The graphs in Figure 1 show that there is a linear relationship between the tension of carbon dioxide in the alveoli and ventilation, and that in most situations carbon dioxide is a stronger stimulus to ventilation than anoxia, which does not stimulate ventilation until the tension of oxygen has fallen to about 7.3 kPa (55 mmHg). The graph also shows that chronic bronchitics of blue bloating type respond less vigorously to carbon dioxide than normals. This is discussed later in the book.

4i   Breathlessness in left ventricular failure

This is due mainly to the lung becoming *stiff* as blood accumulates in the pulmonary vasculature behind the failing ventricle. As a consequence the *work* performed and the *tension* developed by the respiratory muscles increases, and as described in the previous answer leads to the sensation we know as breathlessness.

The process is exacerbated by the hydrostatic pressure at the venous end of the pulmonary capillaries rising to greater values than the oncotic pressure exerted by the plasma proteins. As a consequence fluid is not drawn back into the vasculature at the venous end of the pulmonary capillaries and instead collects in the interstitial space, adding to the stiffness of the lung.

In addition, although mild anoxia does not stimulate respiration, in *severe* left ventricular failure associated with cyanosis, the patient's sense of breathlessness will be compounded by the respiratory centre being stimulated by anoxia brought about by *mismatching of the normally well matched ventilation and perfusion of the lungs, and also by impaired diffusion of oxygen* through any frank oedema within the alveolar and interstitial spaces.

4ii   The patterns of breathlessness associated with left ventricular failure

These may be summarised as follows:
- *Breathlessness on exertion* due to the mechanisms discussed in the preceding paragraphs.
- *Orthopnoea* (breathlessness when lying flat) which is due in part to further pulmonary congestion occurring as a result of

redistribution of fluid from the periphery to the pulmonary circulation when the patient is recumbent, and also in part to the abdominal contents pushing on the diaphragm.

- *Paroxysmal nocturnal dyspnoea* (PND) which is associated with the patient waking from sleep and fighting for breath. PND occurs during REM (rapid eye movement) sleep and is due possibly to venospasm in capacitance vessels during this form of sleep causing blood to move to the pulmonary circulation from areas of pooling in the veins of the limbs and gut.
- *Acute pulmonary oedema* which occurs when the hydrostatic pressure within the pulmonary capillaries rises to more than 25 mmHg and is sufficiently greater than the oncotic pressure exerted by the plasma proteins to cause marked interstitial oedema and the accumulation of free fluid in the alveoli.
- *Wheeze* which is due to narrowing of the airways as a result of mucosal oedema and bronchospasm.

3   Cheyne–Stokes respiration

This is alternating periods of hyperventilation and apnoea due to depression and altered sensitivity to carbon dioxide of the respiratory centre in the brain stem. During the periods of hyperventilation the patient blows off excessive quantities of carbon dioxide causing a lowering of carbon dioxide tension in the blood, loss of carbon dioxide drive to respiration and a period of apnoea during which levels of the gas build up again until they are sufficient to stimulate the next period of hyperventilation.

The main causes of Cheyne-Stokes respiration are stroke and cerebrovascular disease, but it also occurs with cardiac failure.

Cyanosis
Question

6   What is cyanosis? What is central cyanosis and what is peripheral cyanosis? In what conditions do they occur?

Answer

6   Cyanosis

Cyanosis is a purplish/blue discoloration of the skin or mucous membranes due to the presence of unoxygenated haemoglobin, or occasionally other reduced forms of haemoglobin such as methaemoglobin. As with the assessment of many physical signs, the assessment of cyanosis is highly subjective with fairly frequent inter observer disagreements about its presence. Traditionally cyanosis is associated with the presence of at least 5 g of unoxygenated haemoglobin per dl blood. Cyanosis is difficult to detect in the presence of anaemia.

- *Peripheral cyanosis* is due to increased extraction of oxygen in the extremities as a result of stasis caused by peripheral vasoconstriction. Peripheral cyanosis occurs in *cold temperatures, shock, cardiac failure and peripheral vascular disease.*

- *Central cyanosis* is present when the tongue and mucous membranes of the mouth are cyanosed and is due to failure of oxygenation of the blood in the lungs. Central cyanosis is caused by *cardiac failure, respiratory failure, and right to left heart shunts.*

Quality of the pulse

Questions

7 How does a normal pulse differ from an atherosclerotic pulse?

8 In what conditions is a small weak pulse (pulsus parvus) found?

9 In what condition is a slow rising pulse (pulsus tardis) found? To what is it due?

10 To what is a bounding pulse due? In what conditions is a bounding or waterhammer pulse found?

11 In what conditions is a jerky pulse found? To what is it due?

12 What is pulsus alternans? In which condition is it found? From what must it be differentiated?

13 Describe pulsus bisferiens. In what conditions is it found?

14 Describe arterial pulsus paradoxus. How is it measured and by what mechanisms is it thought to be caused? In what conditions is it found?

Answers

7 Normal and atherosclerotic pulses

Normally the radial pulse is soft to palpation. In persons with widespread atherosclerosis it is often firm and less easily compressed.

8 A small weak pulse (pulsus parvus)

This is found in conditions in which the stroke volume is reduced, for example cardiac failure, mitral stenosis, shock or hypovolaemia of any cause.

9 A slow rising pulse (pulsus tardus)

This is found in aortic stenosis and is due to left ventricular systole being prolonged as a result of the mechanical obstruction to outflow associated with this condition.

10 A bounding pulse

This is due to an increased stroke volume, a wide pulse pressure and decreased peripheral resistance and is found in conditions such as anxiety, fever, anaemia, pregnancy, thyrotoxicosis and marked bradycardia.

A similar pulse may also be found in persistent ductus arteriosus and large arteriovenous fistulae, and is due to abnormally rapid run-off of blood from the high pressure systemic arterial system to the relatively low pressure pulmonary artery in persistent ductus, and the low pressure systemic venous system in arteriovenous fistula.

In aortic regurgitation the pulse is also bounding. This is because of the ejection of a large volume of blood into the aorta in early systole and the regurgitation of part of it back into the heart in late systole and diastole. In aortic regurgitation this effect is known as a *waterhammer pulse*, and is most easily demonstrated by assessing the pulse in the patient's *forearm* in the lowered and raised positions with the *palm* of one's own *left* hand. In the lowered position the grip is adjusted until the patient's pulse is just not palpable. Keeping the pressure of one's grip exactly the same, the patient's arm is then lifted with one's own right hand. If the pulse is waterhammer it will produce an easily perceived thud that is similar to the thud produced by the sudden flow of water in a Victorian toy known as a waterhammer—hence the name of the sign.

11   A jerky or thudding pulse of short duration

This is found in severe mitral regurgitation, ventricular septal defect and hypertrophic obstructive cardiomyopathy. In mitral regurgitation and ventricular septal defect this is because as explained on page 188 much of the stroke volume passes *very rapidly* into the low pressure left atrium or right ventricle respectively. In the systemic circulation this rapid flow of blood inside the heart results in a small volume pulse of rapid or jerky quality. In hypertrophic cardiomyopathy the jerky nature of the pulse is due to the flow of blood from the left ventricle being cut off by contraction and obstruction during systole of the outflow tract of the left ventricle.

12   Pulsus alternans

This is characterised by alternate strong and weak beats in the

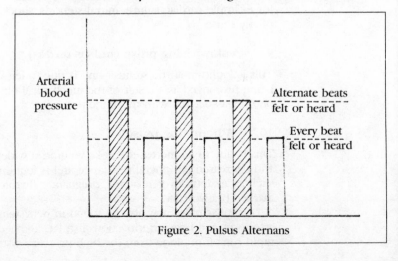

Figure 2. Pulsus Alternans

arterial pulse. It is a sign of left ventricular failure, and is relatively uncommon. Its cause is unknown. In a well developed case it may be detected by palpation of the radial pulse. In less obvious cases it is best detected by monitoring the systolic blood pressure with a sphygmomanometer and either palpating the pulse or listening with a stethoscope. Pulsus alternans has to be differentiated from *pulsus bigeminus (coupling)* in which a normal sinus beat is followed by a ventricular extrasystole that is usually weak and accompanied by a compensatory pause. In pulsus bigeminus the beats therefore occur in pairs followed by a compensatory pause. On the ECG, in pulsus alternans the QRS complexes are all of the same configuration; in pulsus bigeminus sinus beats alternate with ventricular extrasystoles that are usually followed by a compensatory pause.

13   Pulsus bisferiens

This is characterised by two peaks in systole and a mid-systolic dip. It is most easily felt in the carotid arteries. The first peak is known as the percussion wave and is due to left ventricular ejection. The second peak is presumed to be due to a reflected wave from the periphery. Pulsus bisferiens may be found in aortic regurgitation (with or without stenosis), and hypertrophic cardiomyopathy. In the latter condition the mid-systolic dip is due to the obstruction of the outflow tract that occurs after the early part of systole has produced the percussion wave. A reflected wave from the periphery produces the second or tidal wave.

Pulsus bisferiens must be differentiated from *the dicrotic pulse* that is found occasionally in low cardiac output states in which a diminished cardiac output is ejected into a soft elastic aorta. With the dicrotic pulse a second peak occurs during early *diastole* as a result of the aortic valve closing and causing a reflected wave.

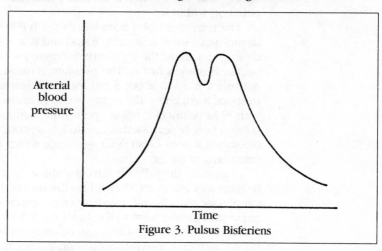

Figure 3. Pulsus Bisferiens

14   The answer to this question is given on page 147.

Jugular venous pulse (JVP)

Questions

15 Why is the internal rather than the external jugular vein usually used in assessment of the JVP? Why is the pressure measured from the sternal angle? What is the pressure in normals? In what conditions is it elevated? In what condition does it rise during inspiration?

16i What are the three wave components of the JVP? To what are they due?

ii What are the two troughs in the JVP? To what are they due?

17 In what way is the JVP different in a patient with atrial fibrillation?

18 List the causes of large waves in the JVP? What is the explanation of large waves in the JVP on the right side of the circulation in conditions of the left side, such as aortic stenosis?

Answers

Examination of the JVP yields information about two parameters, namely (a) the central venous pressure, and (b) the type of wave pattern. By convention clinical examination of the heart and JVP is conducted with the patient lying at an angle of about 45 degrees, although a lower position may be better if the pressure in the jugular vein is low, whilst a higher position may be best in patients in whom the pressure is greatly raised.

15 Measurement of the jugular venous pressure

Because free communication between the superior vena cava and the *external* jugular vein is often interrupted by valves and fascial planes, the internal jugular vein is preferred, although the external jugular vein may be used if there is a free rise and fall and visible pulsation within it.

The reference point from which the JVP is measured is the sternal angle since it is easily found and is at a fixed height of about 5 cm above the right atrium regardless of whether the patient is upright or flat. The pressure is measured vertically. In normals it is up to about 3 cm above the sternal angle, that is up to about 8 cm above the right atrium. Abnormal elevation occurs with right ventricular failure, pericardial tamponade and constriction, hypervolaemia due to intravenous fluid overload, and the superior vena cava (SVC) syndrome which is usually due to carcinoma of the bronchus.

Normally the JVP falls during inspiration as increased quantities of blood are drawn into the thorax. In cardiac tamponade and chronic constrictive pericarditis, however, due to impaired venous return to the heart the JVP often rises paradoxically with inspiration, an observation known as *Kussmaul's sign*. The mechanism underlying this is explained on page 148.

16   The three waves and two troughs of the JVP

i   The three wave components of the JVP are illustrated in Figure 4.

The waves may be explained as follows:

a   is due to right atrial contraction causing a small volume of blood to pass backwards into the great veins;

c   is due to doming and increased protrusion of the tricuspid valve into the right atrium at the beginning of ventricular systole;

v   is due to passive venous return filling the right atrium and great veins whilst the tricuspid valve is closed.

ii   The two troughs in the JVP are explained as follows:

x   is due to a fall in venous pressure as a result of: relaxation of the right atrium during atrial diastole, and downward movement of the tricuspid valve as ventricular systole continues.

y   is due to a fall in venous pressure as the tricuspid valve opens and blood falls through into the right ventricle.

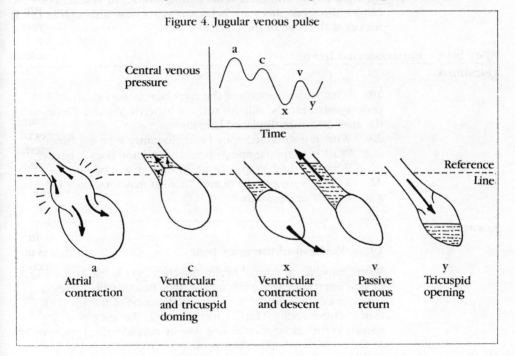

Figure 4. Jugular venous pulse

Central venous pressure

Time

Reference Line

a	c	x	v	y
Atrial contraction	Ventricular contraction and tricuspid doming	Ventricular contraction and descent	Passive venous return	Tricuspid opening

17   The JVP in atrial fibrillation

This consists of only two waves, the c wave and the v wave, as there is no co-ordinated contraction of the atrium to produce an a wave.

18   Large waves in the JVP

These may be due to:

●   *A large a wave*, found in conditions in which increased amounts of blood flow backwards into the great veins as a result of the right atrium contracting against increased resistance. Examples of this are:

a   Tricuspid stenosis.

b   Stiffness and non-compliance of the right ventricle due for instance to right ventricular hypertrophy resulting from pulmonary hypertension or pulmonary stenosis.

c   Bulging of a hypertrophied interventricular septum into the right ventricle as a result of severe *left* ventricular hypertrophy due for instance to aortic stenosis or hypertrophic cardiomyopathy.

●   *Conditions in which the right atrium contracts whilst the tricuspid valve is closed*, for example complete heart block or ventricular tachycardia, or junctional rhythm in which the atria contract during or after rather than before ventricular systole. In this situation the waves are often referred to as *cannon* waves.

●   *Tricuspid regurgitation due to blood regurgitating back into* the right atrium and great veins during ventricular systole. For historical reasons this wave is known as a v wave although in fact it occurs at the time of the c wave.

Apex beat and parasternal heave
Questions

19   What is the position of the apex beat in normal health? In general, what are the relative roles of hypertrophy and dilatation as the apex becomes displaced laterally?

20i   What is a sustained apex beat? How may it be explained?

ii   What is a tapping apex? In what condition does it occur?

21   What is a double apex beat? To what may it be due?

22   What is a parasternal heave? To what may it be due? How is it most easily demonstrated?

Answers

19   Position of the apex beat

When palpable, in normal health the apex beat is felt in the fourth or fifth intercostal space within the mid-clavicular line. Lateral displacement is generally due more to dilatation of the left ventricle than to hypertrophy. Thus in aortic stenosis the apex beat may remain in the mid-clavicular line despite considerable hypertrophy. As the apex moves laterally it is often referred to as being in the anterior axillary line, the mid-axillary line or even the posterior axillary line.

20   Sustained apex and tapping apex

i   *Sustained apex:* normally the apex beat moves out for the first third of systole only, and thereafter retracts. As the heart hypertrophies the outward movement is prolonged giving rise to a *sustained or heaving apex*.

ii   *Tapping apex:* this is due to the velocity of closure of the mitral valve being sufficiently fast to cause a palpable tapping at the apex. It is a sign of mitral stenosis which should therefore be suspected in any patient with a tapping apex. The mechanism underlying it is explained on page 185.

21   Double apex

A double apex, or an apex beat consisting of two components, is an unusual sign. It may be caused by:

● A palpable *atrial impulse* occurring *late in diastole* and preceding the main outward movement of the apex. This type of apex is due to left atrial contraction becoming unusually powerful in response to the resistance to flow offered by conditions such as mitral stenosis, aortic stenosis and hypertrophic cardiomyopathy.

● Bulging *during late systole*, when the apex would normally be retracting, occurs with left ventricular aneurysm.

22   Parasternal heave

This is lifting of the sternum due to an abnormally forceful cardiac impulse. Right ventricular hypertrophy is the commonest cause of a parasternal heave, but occasionally a heaving sternum may result from the great enlargement of the *left* atrium or *left* ventricle associated with severe mitral regurgitation. A parasternal heave is most easily demonstrated by feeling with and watching the heel of the right palm placed on the sternum and using one's extended fingers as a lever to magnify any movement.

Heart sounds

Questions

23   What is the first heart sound due to?

24   The main abnormality of the first heart sound is in its intensity or loudness. Upon what does the loudness of the heart sounds depend? In what conditions is the first heart sound likely to be loud, and in what conditions is it likely to be soft?

25   What is the second heart sound due to?

26   Explain physiological splitting of the second heart sound. What is wide fixed splitting, and what is reversed or paradoxical splitting of the second heart sound? In what conditions are they found?

27   In what conditions is the second heart sound loud? In what conditions is it soft?

28   Describe the third heart sound. How may it be explained? In what conditions is it found?

29   Describe the fourth heart sound. How may it be explained? How is it distinguished from a split first heart sound? In what conditions is it found?

30   Over what areas of the thorax is it best to listen for each of the heart sounds?

Answers

23   The first heart sound (S_1)

This is due to closure of the mitral and tricuspid valves.

24   Intensity of the first heart sound

Although splitting of the first heart sound may occur, for instance in right bundle branch block due to closure of the tricuspid valve being delayed, the main abnormalities of the first heart sound relate to its *intensity or loudness* rather than its timing.

Loudness of the heart sounds depends more upon the *velocity of closure* of the valves than upon the strength of ventricular contraction. S_1 is therefore *loud* in conditions in which cardiac output is high and the pulse fast, for example anxiety, anaemia, hyperthyroidism. It is also loud in mitral stenosis because the high pressure generated in the left atrium in order to push blood through the narrowed valve holds the valve open for longer than normal into the early part of left ventricular systole. A high velocity closure of the valve, causing a loud sound, is then effected by the full force of left ventricular contraction.

The first heart sound is *quiet* in conditions in which the velocity of closure of the valves is low, for example following myocardial infarction, or rheumatic mitral incompetence in which the chordae tendineae have become shortened and so prevent proper closure of the valve, or *advanced* mitral stenosis in which the cusps of the valve have become calcified and immobile.

● Both the first and second heart sounds may be quiet in conditions in which conduction of sounds to the stethoscope are impaired, for instance obesity, emphysema, pericardial effusion or chronic constrictive pericarditis.

25   The second heart sound (S_2)

This is due to closure of the aortic valve (A_2) and the pulmonary valve (P_2).

26   Splitting of the second heart sound

● *Physiological splitting of the second heart sound.* In normals during *expiration* the two valves close at the same time. In *inspiration* there is normally audible splitting of the second sound as more blood is drawn into the thorax and right side of the heart. As a consequence right ventricular systole takes longer which causes delay in closure of the pulmonary valve.

● *Wide fixed splitting of the second heart sound* occurs in atrial septal defect and is due to delayed closure of the pulmonary valve. The mechanism underlying the wide fixed split is the increased flow of blood through the right side of the heart causing right ventricular stroke volume to be increased. As a consequence the time taken for right ventricle systole is increased, causing closure of the pulmonary valve to be delayed.

● *Reversed splitting of the second heart sound* is most easily understood by considering the situation with left bundle branch block. Due to the delayed conduction found in this condition, left ventricular systole is delayed and as a consequence *aortic valve closure is delayed and occurs after the pulmonary valve has closed.* The sequence of events this causes is as follows:

During inspiration the two elements of S_2 are brought together as closure of the pulmonary valve is delayed by the increased amount of blood drawn into the right side of the thorax. During expiration they move apart, which of course is a paradoxical reversal of the normal sequence of events.

Paradoxical or reversed splitting of the second heart sound may also be found in conditions in which left ventricular systole is prolonged mechanically, such as for instance aortic stenosis, hypertension and cardiomyopathy.

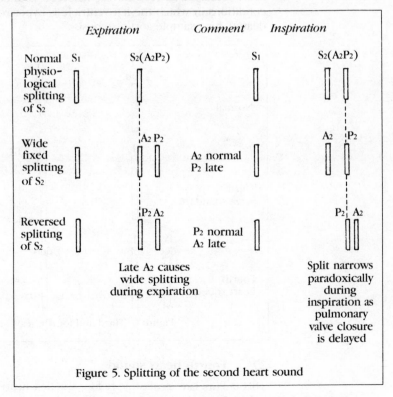

Figure 5. Splitting of the second heart sound

27   Intensity or loudness of the second heart sound

● *A loud S_2* is due to abnormally high pressure causing the valve to shut with greater than normal velocity. As a consequence

A_2 is often loud in systemic hypertension, and P_2 in pulmonary hypertension.

NOTE: As a consequence of both pulmonary hypertension and increased blood flow, in atrial septal defect P_2 may be both loud and widely split.

● A *soft* S_2 occurs in situations in which stiffness of the valves interferes with their closure. As a consequence A_2 is often soft in aortic stenosis, and P_2 in pulmonary stenosis.

28   Third heart sound

When present this occurs shortly after the second heart sound. It may be audible in healthy persons aged under 40, but is a pathological finding in persons aged over about 40. Its cause is unknown, but it occurs in diastole during the period of rapid filling of the ventricles and may be thought of as creaking of a stiff diseased ventricle (usually the left) as it fills. It may be heard after myocardial infarction, in chronic constrictive pericarditis (but not tamponade), mitral regurgitation, and in conditions in which the heart is dilated, such as cardiac failure. It is uncommon in conditions in which the left ventricle is hypertrophied but not dilated, for example aortic stenosis.

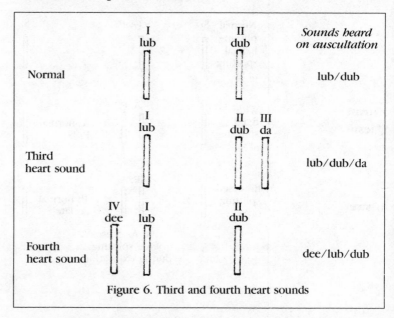

Figure 6. Third and fourth heart sounds

29   Fourth heart sound

This occurs late in diastole before the first heart sound, and is due to atrial contraction squeezing blood from the atrium against a raised end diastolic pressure into an already partially filled diseased stiff left ventricle. In a sense it may therefore also be thought of as the creaking of a diseased stiff ventricle. It is always pathological, and may be heard in ventricular disease of most causes, particularly hypertension and myocardial infarction.

A fourth heart sound has to be distinguished from a split first sound. This can be difficult. However, the first heart sound is *soft* after a fourth sound, whereas the second component of a split first sound is of *normal intensity*.

NOTE: Third and fourth sounds from the right ventricle become louder during inspiration as more blood is drawn into the right side of the heart.

30 Where to listen for each of the heart sounds

● *First heart sound.* Since the first heart sound is due to closure of the mitral and tricuspid valves, it is most easily heard over the areas to which sound from these valves is conducted, that is over the apex and left sternal edge.

● *Second heart sound.* Since the second heart sound is due to closure of the aortic and pulmonary valves, it is most easily heard over the areas to which sound from these valves is conducted, that is over the second right and second left intercostal spaces respectively.

● *Summary.* In normal clinical practice it is therefore best to concentrate on the first heart sound at the apex and left sternal edge, and to ignore the second heart sound in these areas; and to concentrate on the second heart sound in both second intercostal spaces, and to ignore the first heart sound in these areas. Third and fourth heart sounds should be listened for over the ventricles, that is between the apex and left sternal edge.

Murmurs

Questions

31 What is a murmur? What is a thrill?

32 What are the three simple questions that have to be answered in interpreting a murmur?

Answers

31 Definitions

A murmur is an audible vibration produced by the turbulent flow of blood from a narrow to a wider channel. It therefore follows that a murmur is heard best over the point where the channel widens, or beyond the narrowing in the direction in which the blood is flowing.

A thrill is a palpable vibration. A loud murmur may produce a palpable vibration or thrill.

32 Three simple questions to be answered in interpreting a murmur

The interpretation and timing of a murmur, and whether it is a systolic or diastolic, early, mid or late is best accomplished by

asking three simple questions:
- What does it sound like?
- Where is it loudest?
- Where does it radiate to?

- *What does it sound like?* Just as we recognise individual people, animals and cars by the impact of their totality and not by analysing them, so murmurs are recognised. As Sir Thomas Lewis said, murmurs are recognised 'as one learns to know a dog's bark'. Once recognised the timing of a murmur becomes easy.

With the exception of the rare machinery murmur of persistent ductus arteriosus, which is audible throughout the cardiac cycle, *there are only three types of murmur*; systolic murmurs that sound like Sh-sh-sh or occcasionally like a loud coarse Ccr-r-rh; high pitched decrescendo diastolic murmurs that die away like the clash of a pair of cymbals, and sound like TWAaa; and low pitched diastolic rumbles that are best described as an absence of silence, and sound like a very soft Ur-r-rh.

Systolic murmurs are by far the commonest, and may be of variable length, occur at different times in systole, and are classified on a loudness scale of 1–6. Many systolic murmurs are functional and of no clinical significance, but have to be sorted from those that represent serious underlying pathology. Diastolic murmurs are classified on a loudness scale of 1–4.

- *Where is it loudest? Where does it radiate to?*
Using these parameters the interpretation of most murmurs may be summarised as follows:

Character of murmur	Loudest point	Radiation	Diagnosis
Systolic murmurs			
Sh-sh-sh	Apex	Axilla	Mitral regurgitation
Sh-sh-sh	Left sternal edge		Ventricular septal defect Tricuspid regurgitation*
Sh-sh-sh or Ccr-r-rh	Aortic area	Carotids	Aortic stenosis
Sh-sh-sh	Pulmonary area	—	Pulmonary stenosis Atrial septal defect
Diastolic murmurs			
TWAaa	Aortic area	Left sternal edge	Aortic regurgitation Rarely pulmonary regurgitation
Ur-r-rh	Apex	—	Mitral stenosis Rarely the Carey Coombs murmur or Austin Flint murmur
Tr-ar-ah	Left sternal edge	—	Tricuspid stenosis*

* These murmurs increase during inspiration as more blood is drawn into the thorax and right side of the heart.

Auscultation of the chest in cardiac and non-cardiac disease

Questions

33 List the cardiac and non-cardiac causes of the following signs. Explain the mechanisms underlying them.
  i   Reduced/quiet breath sounds
  ii Increased or bronchial breath sounds
34i What are early crackles, and what are late crackles? How may they be explained? In what conditions does each occur?
  ii What is a wheeze? To what is it due? In what conditions does wheezing occur?

Answers

33   Quiet and loud/bronchial breath sounds

During the examination of the chest it is important to judge whether the breath sounds are normal, quiet or loud.

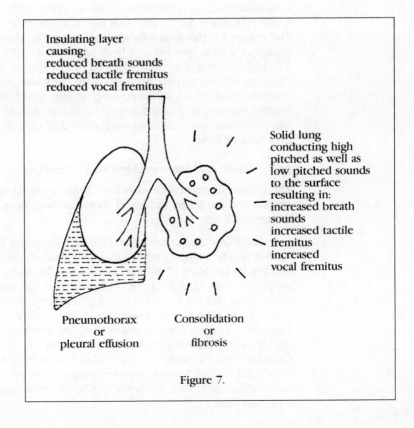

Insulating layer causing:
reduced breath sounds
reduced tactile fremitus
reduced vocal fremitus

Solid lung conducting high pitched as well as low pitched sounds to the surface resulting in:
increased breath sounds
increased tactile fremitus
increased vocal fremitus

Pneumothorax
or
pleural effusion

Consolidation
or
fibrosis

Figure 7.

i   *Quiet or reduced breath sounds* are heard in the following
conditions:

● *Pleural effusion or pneumothorax.* As illustrated, in these
conditions there is an abnormal layer around the lung that
insulates it and keeps it away from the chest wall and so reduces
conduction of the breath sounds to the surface. In addition, as
described in the next paragraph, the breath sounds are also
reduced in these conditions by the collapse of the lung with which
they are associated.

● *Collapse of part or whole of a lung.* In this condition less air
flows in and out of the lung than normal, and so less sound is
conducted.

● *Chronic obstructive airways disease*, and quite separately
diseases associated with a reduction of vital capacity such as the
Guillain–Barré syndrome, polio and ankylosing spondylitis. Due to
obstruction of the airways in chronic obstructive airways disease,
and reduced movements of the chest wall in conditions associated
with reduction of vital capacity, the flow of air in and out of the
lungs is reduced in each of these examples, resulting in the
conduction of less sound.

ii   *Loud/bronchial or increased breath sounds* are heard in
conditions such as consolidation due to pneumonia or gross
localised fibrosis due to previous tuberculosis or bronchiectasis.
The reason for this is as follows. The flow of air through the larynx
produces a wide spectrum of both high and low pitched sounds.
The high pitched sounds are filtered out by normal lung and as a
consequence normal breath sounds are fairly low pitched. By
contrast 'solid' or consolidated lung conducts both high and low
pitched sounds. As a consequence the breath sounds are louder
and palpation more resonant over an area of consolidation than
over normal lung.

34   Early and late crackles and wheezing

The terms râle and crepitation have been replaced by the term
crackle and the terms rattle and rhonchus have been replaced by
the term wheeze.

i   *Early and late crackles:* crackles are explosive popping
sounds due to snapping open of airways, and not as was previously
thought to bubbling of air through fluid in the lungs. Airways
supplying easily distensible or compliant parts of the lungs open
earlier than airways to stiff non-compliant parts. The timing of
crackles can therefore be used in assessing underlying pathology.
Crackles occurring *early* in inspiration are an unusual sign of
asthma, emphysema and chronic obstructive airways disease.
Crackles occurring *towards the end of or late* in inspiration are
associated with stiff non-compliant lungs due to conditions such as
*left ventricular failure, pulmonary fibrosis, consolidation and
bronchiectasis*.

ii   *A wheeze* is any continuous sound, and is due to the reed-like effect of the opposed walls of a narrowed bronchus oscillating as air flows through it. Wheezes are heard in chronic obstructive airways disease, asthma and occasionally in left ventricular failure.

Pleural effusion
Questions

35   List the signs of pleural effusion.
36   Define the terms 'transudate' and 'exudate'. What are the changes or processes in the capillaries that give rise to each? List the causes of pleural effusion, classifying them as either a transudate or an exudate.
37   List the main causes of blood-stained pleural effusion.

Answers

35   Signs of pleural effusion

When examining any part of the body it is important to proceed in a proper disciplined order. In this way nothing is overlooked. When examining the chest the proper order in which to proceed is inspection, palpation, percussion, and lastly auscultation. Using this order, the signs of pleural effusion may be stated as:
● *On inspection* the affected side of the chest usually moves less than the normal side. This is because an effusion causes collapse of the adjacent part of the lung. As a consequence less air flows in and out and the chest wall moves less.
● *On palpation* the trachea is deviated away from an effusion of any size. This is because an effusion pushes the lung towards the opposite side of the chest. In addition, as explained in the answer to question 33, tactile fremitus is reduced.
● *On percussion* the fluid, being dense, causes a 'solid' or stony dull note.
● *On auscultation* the breath sounds and vocal fremitus are reduced for the reasons explained in the answer to question 33.

36   Causes and classification of pleural effusion

Transudate: an effusion containing < 25 grams protein per litre, due either to increased hydrostatic pressure or decreased oncotic pressure at the venous end of the pleural capillaries.

Examples

● Left ventricular failure
● Hypoproteinaemia of any cause (see page 151)

Exudate: an effusion containing > 30 grams protein per litre, due to conditions causing the pleural capillaries to be more permeable to protein than normal.

Examples

● Infections such as bacterial or viral pneumonia or tuberculosis
● Carcinoma of the bronchus
● Pulmonary infarction due most commonly to pulmonary embolus
● Inflammatory conditions involving the pleura, such as rheumatoid arthritis or rheumatic fever
● Abscess, either within the thorax or subdiaphragmatic
● Asbestosis
● A rare manifestation of hypothyroidism
● Meigs' syndrome (association of pleural effusion of unknown aetiology and fibroma of the ovary)

37   The causes of pleural effusion that may be blood stained

● Carcinoma of the bronchus
● Mesothelioma
● Tuberculosis
● Pulmonary infarction
● Trauma
● Ruptured thoracic aortic aneurysm

Further Reading

Braunwald E (ed) (1984). *Heart Disease*, 2nd edition. WB
      Saunders, Philadelphia. Chapters 1, the history; 2, the physical
      examination.

Chapter 2
Cardiac Failure

Definitions; pathophysiology (i)
Questions

1 Define the term 'cardiac failure'.

2i Define the term 'cardiac output'. What are the two parameters that may be multiplied to measure cardiac output?

ii Define the term 'cardiac index'.

3i What is the approximate range, in litres per minute, of the cardiac output in a healthy adult at rest? To what might it rise during exercise?

ii To what sort of levels, in litres per minute, is the cardiac output likely to fall in a patient with heart failure due for instance to generalised ischaemic heart disease?

4 List three of four conditions in which heart failure might be associated with an elevated or high cardiac output. What is the mechanism in each case?

5 Define the term 'stroke volume'. What are the three parameters that determine stroke volume? What is the stroke volume likely to be in a healthy adult at rest?

6 Define the term 'ejection fraction'. What is the ejection fraction likely to be in a healthy adult at rest? To what sort of level might it fall in a case of severe heart failure?

Answers

1 Cardiac failure

Cardiac failure is defined as failure of the pumping action of the heart to maintain the cardiac output at a sufficient level to meet the metabolic needs of the body.

2 Cardiac output and cardiac index

i Cardiac output is defined as the quantity of blood delivered to the systemic circulation per unit of time, and is generally expressed in litres per minute. Cardiac output is the product of stroke volume × heart rate.

ii Cardiac index is the cardiac output related to body size, and is expressed in litres/minute/square metre of body surface area.

3 Cardiac output in a healthy adult and in heart failure

i The cardiac output in a healthy adult at rest is between 4 and

8 litres per minute. During exercise it may rise to about 30 litres per minute in a trained athlete.

ii   In cardiac failure the resting cardiac output may fall as low as 1-3 litres per minute.

4   Cardiac failure with normal or elevated cardiac output

Although the cardiac output is usually low in heart failure due to conditions such as ischaemic heart disease, it may be normal or elevated in heart failure due to conditions in which there is either a central or peripheral decrease in resistance to the flow of blood. Examples of these conditions are:

● *Atrial or ventricular septal defect*, or arteriovenous fistula (A-V shunt) of the type found occasionally in Paget's disease. In these examples the decrease of resistance is *central*.

● *Thyrotoxicosis or fever*. In these examples the decrease of resistance is due to dilatation of *peripheral* arterioles, the resulting increase in cardiac output being part of a generalised response of the body to its increased metabolic needs. A similar mechanism applies in *anaemia*, and is due to a generalised response of the body to the reduced oxygen carrying capacity of the blood.

5   Stroke volume

This is defined as the volume of blood ejected into the systemic circulation with each heart beat. Stroke volume is dependent upon the extent of myocardial fibre shortening, and may be calculated by subtracting the volume of the heart at the end of systole (end systolic volume) from the volume of the heart when it is full of blood at the end of diastole (end diastolic volume).

The three parameters that determine stroke volume are:
● The volume of blood entering the heart (preload).
● The inherent strength of the heart muscle (inherent contractility).
● Resistance to the ejection of blood from the heart during systole (afterload).

Each of these parameters is defined and discussed in the next section. In a healthy adult at rest the stroke volume is between 50 and 90 ml.

6   Ejection fraction

This is defined as the fraction of the contents of the left ventricle when it is full at the end of the diastole that is ejected during systole. It is therefore the difference between the left ventricular end diastolic and end systolic volumes, expressed as a fraction of the diastolic volume. Thus if the end diastolic volume is 140 ml and the end systolic volume is 50 ml, the stroke volume is 90 ml and the ejection fraction 90/140 = 64%. In healthy adults the ejection fraction is 60-70%. In severe cardiac failure it may fall to 10-20%.

Definitions; pathophysiology (ii)
Questions

7   Define the term 'preload'. Expand your answer to include an account of the Frank-Starling hypothesis and its effect on the normal, the failing and the normal exercising heart.
8   Define the term 'inherent contractility'. What happens to inherent contractility in cardiac failure and in the normal exercising heart?
9   Define the term 'afterload'. List the factors that contribute to afterload. Include in your answer an explanation of the law of Laplace? How does it affect afterload?

Answers

7   Preload

This is defined as the force stretching the muscle fibres of the heart when it is resting and full of blood at the end of diastole. It is important because within certain limits the force developed during the contraction of any muscle is related to the initial length of its fibres at rest, which in turn is related to the force stretching them. In the case of the heart the relationship between the force of contraction and the resting length of the muscle fibres is termed

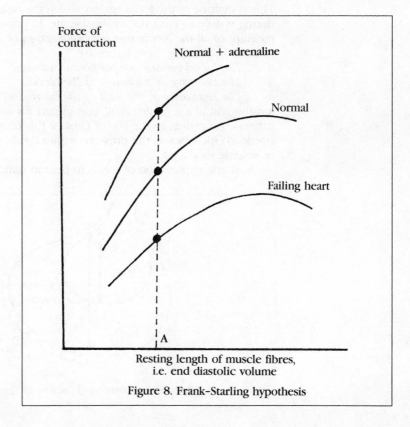

Figure 8. Frank-Starling hypothesis

the *Frank-Starling* mechanism, the implications of which are illustrated in Figure 8.

The relationship shows that:

● At any given end diastolic volume, A, the failing heart develops less force than the normal heart.

● Within certain limits the force of contraction increases as the end diastolic volume increases. Thus as the failing heart dilates it tends to regain some of its power of contraction.

● During exercise, adrenaline increases the power of contraction of the normal heart.

8   The inherent contractility of the cardiac muscle

This is its inherent quality or strength. In cardiac failure this inherent contractility is reduced as a result of disease of the muscle. In the normal heart it is increased during exercise due mainly to adrenaline and the sympathetic nervous system and not to increase in the length of the muscle fibres as might be expected from the Frank-Starling hypothesis. Indeed during exercise the size of the normal heart is either unchanged or even slightly decreased as a result of more complete emptying during systole.

9   Afterload

This is defined as the force against which the heart has to contract during systole to eject the stroke volume. In principle it is a measure of all the forces that oppose ejection of the stroke volume. In practice these forces are:

● *The blood pressure or peripheral resistance.*

● *The viscosity or stickiness of the blood.*

● *The resistance in the wall of the heart itself,* that is the tension within the cardiac wall, due in part for instance to its stiffness. According to the law of *Laplace* this tension (and so afterload) increases as the pressure within the heart and its radius or volume increases.

A simple explanation of this is to bear in mind that force =

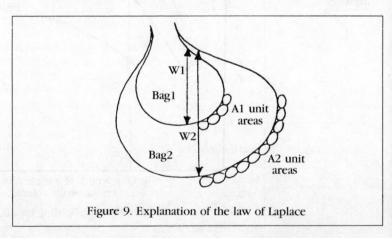

Figure 9. Explanation of the law of Laplace

pressure (force per unit area) × area, and to think of the heart as a bag filled with fluid. If the volume of the bag is increased two important consequences follow as illustrated in Figure 9.

● The weight or *pressure* exerted by the fluid on the walls of Bag 2 is greater than on the walls of Bag 1 because the column of fluid W2 is heavier than the column of fluid W1

● The *area* over which the increased pressure is applied is greater for Bag 2 than for Bag 1. Therefore the *force* exerted on the walls of the two bags by the fluid within each of them is greater for the large bag (Bag 2) than for the small bag (Bag 1) because W2 × A2 (pressure × area) is greater than W1 × A1. Thus when a given volume of fluid is ejected from each bag greater force and work is necessary to eject it from Bag 2 than from Bag 1.

This simple explanation tells only part of the story. In strict mathematical terms the area of a sphere is related to the fourth power of its radius (r^4), so that within a fluid filled sphere the area over which the fluid exerts its pressure is a function of the fourth power of the radius of the sphere, which greatly magnifies the effect of varying the radius.

The implication of this is that afterload for a dilated heart is greater than for a heart of normal size, which of course tends to counteract the beneficial effect of the Frank-Starling hypothesis according to which, as stated on page 30, the failing heart tends to regain some of its power of contraction as it dilates.

Cardiac hypertrophy and dilatation; fluid retention

Questions

10   Explain the *mechanisms* by which the heart (i) hypertrophies, (ii) dilates. What is the upper limit of normal end diastolic pressure?

11   Explain the terms (i) 'forward' and (ii) 'backward' failure used to explain the fluid retention found in heart failure.

Answers

10   **Mechanisms of cardiac hypertrophy and dilatation**

i   *Cardiac hypertrophy:* just as any muscle that is required to work continuously against an increased load responds to the increased metabolic demands made of it by hypertrophying, so the heart hypertrophies in response to a chronic increase of pressure within its walls. This increase of pressure may occur in two main ways:

● *Increased afterload* as found in systemic hypertension or aortic stenosis.

● *Increased preload and end diastolic pressure* as found in heart failure due to aortic regurgitation, mitral regurgitation or ischaemic heart disease. The mechanism underlying the increase of preload and end diastolic pressure is explained in the following paragraph.

ii   *Cardiac dilatation:* as heart failure develops the ventricle fails to empty properly and fails to pump on all the blood it receives. As illustrated, this results in blood being dammed back, causing an increase in the weight or pressure of the column of blood filling the heart, that is an increase in the preload and end diastolic pressure within the heart. The increased filling pressure stretches the walls of the heart, and over a period of time causes them to dilate in much the same way as a balloon dilates as it is blown up.

In normals the end diastolic pressure of the left ventricle is less than 12 mmHg; in left sided heart failure, due to the increased weight of the column of blood filling the heart, it is greater than 12 mmHg.

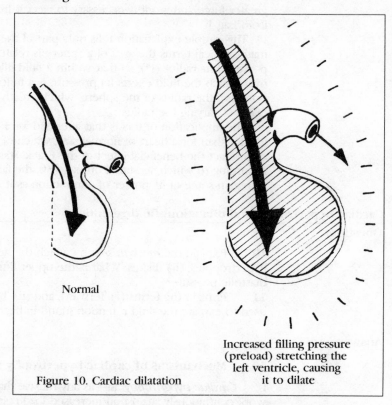

Normal

Increased filling pressure
(preload) stretching the
left ventricle, causing
it to dilate

Figure 10. Cardiac dilatation

11   The fluid retention of heart failure

i   The concept of *forward failure* was propounded by MacKenzie in 1913. At the centre of this concept is the poor perfusion of the kidney that occurs as a consequence of the low cardiac output associated with heart failure. In response to poor perfusion the kidney retains increased amounts of sodium and fluid by the following mechanisms:

• Decrease of glomerular filtration rate that leads to a decrease of sodium and water loss.

• Increased renin production stimulating aldosterone secretion and causing sodium, and as a consequence, water retention.

In addition the load on the heart and so its tendency to forward failure is increased by other counterproductive factors that affect an increase of peripheral resistance. These mechanisms are:

●   Increased sympathetic tone of arterioles.

●   Increased renin production causing formation of angiotensin and further arteriolar constriction.

ii   The concept of *backward failure* was propounded by James Hope in 1832. According to this concept fluid retention occurs because the failing ventricle is unable to pump on all the blood presented to it, that is blood is dammed back behind the failing ventricle as illustrated in Figure 11.

In practice fluid retention is due to a combination of both forward and backward failure, although in situations such as pulmonary oedema of sudden onset, due for instance to myocardial infarction, congestion of the lungs will be due mainly to backward failure since insufficient time will have elapsed for forward failure to have occurred.

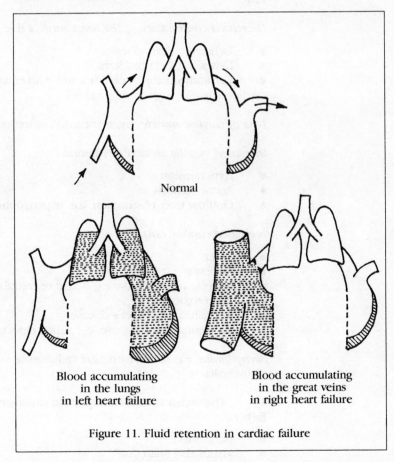

Normal

Blood accumulating
in the lungs
in left heart failure

Blood accumulating
in the great veins
in right heart failure

Figure 11. Fluid retention in cardiac failure

Causes of cardiac failure
Questions

12   List the several *underlying mechanisms* by which the heart
may fail such as, for instance, loss of cardiac muscle. Give examples
of each.
13   List the main *individual specific* causes of left ventricular
failure such as hypertension, myocardial infarction, etc.
14   List the main *individual specific* causes of right ventricular
failure.
15   Cardiomyopathy is one of the underlying causes of heart
failure. Define the term cardiomyopathy. How are the
cardiomyopathies classified? Write a few lines about the way each
class of cardiomyopathy affects the function of the heart.

Answers

**12   The underlying mechanisms by which the heart may
fail**

Decreased contractility of the heart muscle due to:

●   Ischaemic heart disease.
●   Drugs, e.g. beta blockers.
●   Cardiomyopathy. A classification with examples of
cardiomyopathy is given on page 36.

Loss of cardiac muscle, e.g. myocardial infarction.

Increased systolic tension or afterload

●   Hypertension
●   Aortic stenosis
●   Outflow tract obstruction, e.g. hypertrophic cardiomyopathy

Increased cardiac output

●   Fever
●   Anaemia
●   Valvular regurgitation, e.g. aortic or mitral regurgitation
●   Thyrotoxicosis
●   A-V fistula, e.g. Paget's disease
●   Congenital heart disease, e.g. septal defects

Arrhythmias, e.g. supraventricular tachycardia, ventricular
tachycardia.

**13   The main individual specific causes of left ventricular
failure**

●   Ischaemia †
●   Myocardial infarction*
●   Hypertension*

- Valvular heart disease*
- Arrhythmias*
- Drugs, e.g. beta blockers*
- Congenital heart disease*
- Thyrotoxicosis*
- Anaemia*
- Fever*
- Poisons, e.g. alcohol*
- Fistulae, e.g. Paget's disease*
- Vitamin deficiency, e.g. beriberi, due to deficiency of thiamine, vitamin B_1*
- Hypertrophic cardiomyopathy (HOCM)*
- Infiltrations such as amyloid, sarcoidosis and scleroderma
- Rheumatic fever*
- Infective, e.g. cardiomyopathy due to Coxsackie B virus
- Infective endocarditis*

Comment

The importance of seeking a reversible or potentially treatable cause of cardiac failure is amply demonstrated by the following case.

Mr G-B, a 48 year old guest house proprietor, was admitted to hospital with fast atrial fibrillation and a 6 week history of severe cardiac failure. Previously he had been well. There was no past history of hypertension, or evidence of myocardial infarction, valvular disease or other identifiable cause for his heart failure. He admitted to smoking 15 cigarettes and to consuming two to three pints of beer per day. Despite full medical treatment with diuretics, digoxin and vasodilators, his condition worsened in hospital, and after about 6 weeks he was transferred to a cardiac unit for consideration of heart transplantation. A diagnosis of congestive cardiomyopathy was made and his need for a heart transplant accepted. However, whilst awaiting a suitable donor his condition began slowly but continuously to improve until by the end of 6 months he was off all medication, in sinus rhythm, and able to jog 2-3 miles without any difficulty. Only then did he admit that he had not been truthful about his alcohol intake, and that before his hospitalisation he had consumed one bottle of wine, six or seven pints of beer and three large whiskies every day for several years. In retrospect it therefore seemed that he had been suffering from alcoholic cardiomyopathy.

Apart from illustrating the importance of seeking a reversible cause of heart failure, this case also demonstrates how notoriously unreliable heavy drinkers often are about their alcohol consumption.

---

† largely preventable by manipulation of the risk factors listed on page 111.
* potentially treatable provided the disease is not too extensive and has not progressed too far.

14   The main individual specific causes of right ventricular failure

Pulmonary artery hypertension due to:
- Left ventricular failure
- Lung disease, e.g. chronic bronchitis
- Mitral stenosis
- Pulmonary embolus—massive or chronic
- Pulmonary stenosis
- Atrial or ventricular septal defect
- Schistosomiasis

The mechanisms causing pulmonary hypertension in most of the above conditions are discussed on page 200.

15   Cardiomyopathy

This is defined as disease of the muscle fibres of the heart that is not due to ischaemia, hypertension, valvular or congenital heart disease. The condition may be primary, or secondary to virus infection, chronic alcohol poisoning, beriberi, and infiltrations such as amyloidosis, haemachromatosis and sarcoidosis.

Classification

Three types of cardiomyopathy are recognised:
- *Dilated cardiomyopathy* is a syndrome characterised by cardiac enlargement and congestive cardiac failure, frequently with arrhythmias. Functionally the main problem with this type of cardiomyopathy is impaired pumping action of the heart. The condition may be primary or secondary to conditions such as alcohol abuse, beriberi and Coxsackie B virus infection.
- *Obstructive cardiomyopathy*, often known as hypertrophic cardiomyopathy (HOCM), is a primary condition of unknown aetiology characterised by hypertrophy of the walls of the heart, particularly the upper part of the interventricular septum. Functionally this form of cardiomyopathy is associated with small ventricular cavities, stiff ventricular walls and difficulty with filling of the heart, and obstruction of the outflow tract of the left ventricle that in some ways resembles aortic stenosis. Obstructive cardiomyopathy may be complicated by anginal pain, syncope, arrhythmias, heart failure and sudden death.
- *Restrictive cardiomyopathy* is a condition caused by fibrosis of the myocardium or endocardium. As a consequence the walls of the ventricles are rigid and ventricular filling is impaired. The pumping action of the heart and ventricular emptying are well preserved, and in many respects the condition resembles constrictive pericarditis. Restrictive cardiomyopathy occurs mainly in the tropics and is rare in the West, and may be primary, or secondary to amyloidosis.

Symptoms and signs
Questions

16   What are the main symptoms of congestive cardiac failure? Explain the reduced exercise tolerance and the fatigue associated with cardiac failure.

17   What are the main signs of cardiac failure? What are the factors that contribute to cardiac cachexia?

Answers

16   The main symptoms of congestive cardiac failure

These follow from the reduced cardiac output and fluid retention associated with the condition. Congestion of the lungs may lead to *breathlessness* on exertion, orthopnoea (breathlessness on lying flat), paroxysmal nocturnal dyspnoea or frank pulmonary oedema. Full details of the clinical features of these abnormal patterns of breathing and the mechanisms underlying them are given on page 9 in the section on symptoms and signs in cardiac disease. Congestion of the systemic veins may lead to *swelling of the legs and even the trunk*. Details of the mechanism underlying this are given on page 6. The mechanism underlying the *nocturia* associated with cardiac failure is discussed on page 5.

In addition patients with cardiac failure may complain of *pain in the right hypochondrium* due to stretching of the liver capsule as a result of congestion of the liver, *weight loss* due to cardiac cachexia, and *loss of appetite and change of bowel habit* due in part to congestion and poor perfusion of the gastrointestinal tract.

The *reduced exercise tolerance* associated with cardiac failure is due to inability to increase cardiac output with exercise in the same way as normals. *Fatigue* is probably due to an oxygen debt resulting from the blood supply to the muscles and other tissues being insufficient for their needs.

17   The signs of congestive cardiac failure

As details of most of the signs associated with cardiac failure are discussed on pages 10–25 in the section on symptoms and signs in cardiac disease, for the most part they are only summarised here.

The patient may appear *dyspnoeic at rest* and *centrally cyanosed*. The pulse may be of a *small volume* and either *regular or irregular*. Apart from extrasystoles, *atrial fibrillation* is the commonest arrhythmia associated with cardiac failure.

●   Particularly with left ventricular failure, as a result of cardiac dilatation and hypertrophy the *apex beat may be displaced laterally and sustained*. On auscultation of the heart, a *third or fourth heart sound* may be audible or a *murmur* heard reflecting valvular dysfunction. In the lungs, congestion may result in *late inspiratory crackles* or *signs of pleural effusion*.

●   With right ventricular failure, due to fluid retention in the systemic veins, the main signs are *oedema* of dependent parts, *elevation of the jugular venous pulse, hepatomegaly* and occasionally *ascites*. A *parasternal heave* may be felt, reflecting right ventricular hypertrophy.

Cardiac cachexia is due to various factors that include loss of appetite, unreliable absorption of food, poor perfusion of the tissues, diversion of energy to the work of breathing, the increased oxygen and energy requirements of the hypertrophied heart, and sometimes the suppressant effect of digitalis upon the appetite.

Investigation
Questions

18   What are the main abnormalities likely to be seen on the chest x-ray of a patient with well developed left ventricular failure?
19   What are the main abnormalities likely to be seen on an ECG of a patient with left ventricular failure?
20   Which parts of the heart does echocardiography give information about? What is the main indication for echocardiography in cardiac failure?
21   What is left ventricular scintigraphy? How does it differ from thallium scintigraphy? What is the main information that may be gained in cases of cardiac failure by left ventricular scintigraphy?

Answers

18   Chest x-ray

The main abnormalities likely to be seen on a plain chest x-ray are:
●   *Cardiomegaly*—that is an increase on the x-ray of the transverse diameter of the heart, usually assessed as a *relative increase* in the diameter of the heart to more than half the transverse diameter of the thorax, although it may be assessed *absolutely* since in more than 95% of normal persons the diameter of the heart is less than 15.5 cm.
It is important to appreciate that the ventricle which is enlarged cannot be accurately determined on a plain chest x-ray.
●   *Prominence of the upper lobe veins*—due to the increased pulmonary venous pressure associated with left ventricular failure causing a relative diversion of blood from the lower to the upper zones in the erect position. This sign is often likened to a stag's horns.
●   *Enlargement of the hila and a ground glass appearance of the perihilar region*. Often this is likened to a bat's wing. It is due to frank pulmonary oedema or rarely, uraemic lung.
●   *Septal lines* which are fine dense lines thought to be due to oedema in lymphatics. Most commonly they are seen in the costophrenic angles. When horizontal they are known as Kerley B lines.
●   *Pleural effusion*.
●   *Calcification in a valve* such as the aortic valve may be seen occasionally, more especially on a lateral film.

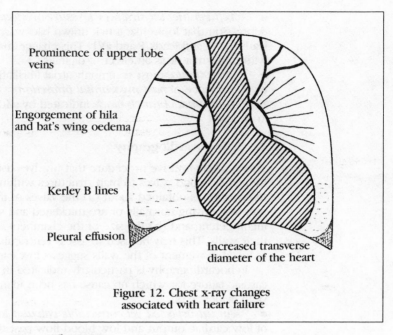

Prominence of upper lobe
veins

Engorgement of hila
and bat's wing oedema

Kerley B lines

Pleural effusion

Increased transverse
diameter of the heart

Figure 12. Chest x-ray changes
associated with heart failure

19   The ECG

This may be normal despite severe left ventricular failure.
However, the following changes may be seen.

- *Left ventricular hypertrophy* inferred when addition of the
depth of the S wave in lead V_1, and the height of the R wave in
lead V_6 is greater than 35 mm (S in V_1 + R in V_6 > 35 mm).

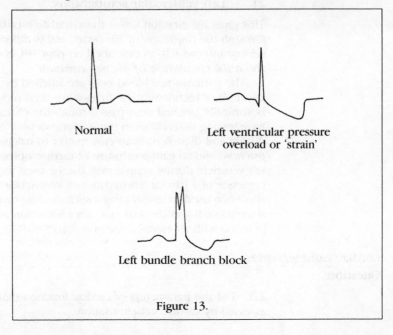

Normal

Left ventricular pressure
overload or 'strain'

Left bundle branch block

Figure 13.

- *Left ventricular strain or pressure overload* suggested by ST depression that looks like a tick drawn backwards in the lateral leads V4–V6 and leads 1 and aV1. This change may also be seen with ischaemia or as an effect of digitalis.
- *Arrhythmia*, most commonly atrial fibrillation.
- Evidence of *past myocardial infarction*.
- *Left bundle branch block* indicated by wide QRS complexes in all leads.

20   Echocardiography

This is a non-invasive procedure that involves using ultra high frequency sound waves to map structures within the heart. Information is obtained about (a) the valves of the heart, whether they are moving normally or are thickened and stenosed or incompetent, and (b) the size of the chambers and movements of their walls. This may be used to assess ventricular function since reduced movement of the walls suggests low cardiac output.

Echocardiography is particularly indicated in patients with cardiac failure for which no cause has been identified as it may yield evidence of:
- *An unsuspected yet correctable valvular lesion* that because of low cardiac output and low blood flow past the valve is not producing an audible murmur.
- *An unsuspected cardiac aneurysm* identified by abnormal outward movement of the ventricular wall during systole.
- *Obstructive cardiomyopathy* suggested by thickening of the ventricular septum.

21   Left ventricular scintigraphy

This gives information about the circulation of blood as it flows *through the chambers of the heart*, and is different to thallium scintigraphy which, as described on page 98, gives information about *the circulation of the myocardium*.

The patient's red blood cells are labelled by an intravenous injection of technetium-99. Images are then recorded as the isotopically labelled cells pass through the chambers of the heart. By assessing differences in the size and density of images taken in systole and diastole it is an easy matter to calculate *the ejection fraction*, and so gain a measure of cardiac output. Bulging of the left ventricle during systole may also be used to assess the presence of a cardiac aneurysm. Left ventricular scintigraphy has also been used to assess prognosis following myocardial infarction, since mortality in the first year after infarction is greatly increased in those with an ejection fraction <40%.

Cardiac catheterisation
Question

22i   List the parameters of cardiac function that may be assessed by cardiac catheterisation.

ii Briefly describe the different methods or techniques of cardiac catheterisation.

iii State the Fick principle of measuring cardiac output.

iv What are the main indications for catheterising each side of the heart in patients with heart failure?

Answer

22i The parameters of cardiac function that may be assessed by cardiac catheterisation

Passage of a catheter through the heart may be used to obtain information about:

- The anatomy of a lesion
- The physiology or severity of a lesion
- Cardiac output
- Cardiac biopsy and histology

22ii Techniques of cardiac catheterisation

- *Angiography* is the most commonly used method of cardiac catheterisation and involves imaging contrast medium injected into a large vessel or chamber of the heart. It gives information about both the anatomy and the severity of cardiac lesions.

The *route* taken by the medium gives information about the *anatomy* of a lesion, and the *amount and density* of contrast medium that passes an obstruction such as a stenosed coronary artery or aortic valve, passages abnormally across a septal defect, regurgitates backwards into the left ventricle or left atrium with aortic or mitral regurgitation, or fills an aneurysmal sac of the left ventricle gives information about the *severity* of a lesion.

- *Observation of the course taken by the catheter* may give information about the anatomy of a lesion. Examples are passage of the catheter across a septal defect, or along an anomalous pulmonary venous system draining into the *right* side of the heart.

- *Measurement of oxygen saturation on the right side of the heart*. This may provide evidence of a left to right shunt. Thus an increase of oxygen saturation in the right ventricle as a catheter is withdrawn from the pulmonary artery indicates a ventricular septal defect, whilst an increase in the right atrium indicates an atrial septal defect.

- *Pressure measurements*. The severity of a lesion may also be assessed by measurement of either the absolute pressure within a large vessel or chamber of the heart, or by measurement of the pressure gradient across a valve.

Thus for instance, the pressure within the left ventricle at the end of diastole may be measured to assess left ventricular function. In normals it is less than 12 mmHg; in left ventricular failure it is greater than 12 mmHg. Similarly the severity of aortic stenosis may be assessed by measuring the pressure difference between the left ventricle and aorta during systole. A difference greater than 50–60 mmHg indicates severe disease.

- *Cardiac biopsy*. Endocardial biopsy of either the left or the right ventricle is occasionally performed in the diagnosis of cardiomyopathy, and to detect rejection following cardiac transplantation.
- *Measurement of cardiac output*. The oxygen content of central venous blood taken by catheter from the pulmonary artery or outflow tract of the right ventricle may be compared with the oxygen content of arterial blood, and the difference used, as explained below, to calculate the cardiac output by the Fick principle.

22iii   The Fick principle of measuring cardiac output

This states that:

$$\begin{array}{c}\text{Total quantity} \\ \text{oxygen taken up} \\ \text{by the lungs per} \\ \text{minute}\end{array} = \text{cardiac output} \times \left(\begin{array}{c}\text{arterial} \\ \text{oxygen} \\ \text{content}\end{array} - \begin{array}{c}\text{central} \\ \text{venous} \\ \text{oxygen} \\ \text{content}\end{array}\right)$$

This is most easily understood by considering the following diagram (Figure 14), in which □ is the volume of oxygen taken up by each millilitre of blood (the A-V difference) as it passes through the lungs.

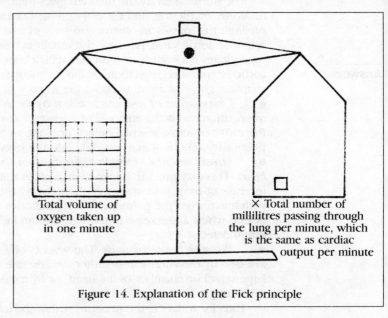

Figure 14. Explanation of the Fick principle

22iv   Indications for cardiac catheterisation in cardiac failure

- *Left heart catheterisation*. Now that most important valvular lesions may be diagnosed by non-invasive means such as echocardiography the main indication for left heart catheterisation in cardiac failure is as a *preoperative procedure* to confirm and quantify the results of non-invasive procedures, and to assess the state of the coronary arteries.

● *Right heart catheterisaton* in heart failure is indicated mainly for the measurement of pulmonary wedge pressure in patients with cardiac failure following myocardial infarction as it allows an informed approximation of events in the *left* atrium and on the *left* side of the heart, and close monitoring of the needs for and responses to therapy without the inherent dangers of catheterising the high pressure left side of the heart.

The pulmonary wedge pressure is measured by wedging the tip of a catheter in a branch of the pulmonary artery so that the vessel is blocked. The pressure measured via the catheter then approximates to the back pressure from the left side of the heart.

Treatment
Questions

23   What are the four cardinal principles of the treatment of cardiac failure?
24   What advice would you give about rest to a patient with congestive cardiac failure?
25   What advice would you give about salt and water intake to a patient with cardiac failure?
26   What are the three types or groups of diuretic used in the treatment of cardiac failure? What are their modes and sites of action? What are the main side effects of each group?

Answers

23   The four cardinal principles of the treatment of cardiac failure

● Search for and if possible *correct any underlying cause.* A list of underlying causes is given on pages 34-35.
● *Reduce the work of the heart* by
a   restricting activity, and
b   if necessary, administering drugs that reduce afterload and preload.
● *Control the excessive salt and water retention* that accompanies cardiac failure.
● Enhance myocardial contractility *by administering digitalis if indicated*, or other drugs such as dopamine or xamoterol.

24   Advice about rest

The degree to which activity should be restricted depends upon the severity of the condition and the individual patient's needs. Advice may vary from slight reduction of activity to rest at home for weeks or months.

25   Salt and water intake

● *Salt intake.* With the advent of effective modern diuretics there is usually no longer a need for unpalatable strict salt restriction. Nonetheless in cases in which it is difficult to control cardiac failure with drugs alone, advice should be given to avoid commercially prepared fast foods which are often rich in salt, and also to avoid adding salt at table.

● *Water intake.* Generally restriction of water is not necessary; however, occasionally in an advanced case of cardiac failure the patient may be unable to excrete a water load and as a consequence may develop dilutional hyponatraemia. In this situation restriction of water intake to 750–1000 ml per day for a period may be helpful.

26   Diuretics: the three main types used in the treatment of cardiac failure

● *Thiazides*, for example chlorothiazide 0.5–1 g daily, hydrochlorothiazide 25–100 mg daily and bendrofluazide 2.5–10 mg daily.

Thiazides act by inhibiting the reabsorption of sodium and chloride ions from the part of the renal tubule just proximal to the distal tubule. Some of the unabsorbed sodium is subsequently absorbed in the distal tubule where it is exchanged for potassium and hydrogen ions which pass out in the urine. As a consequence thiazides may cause *hypokalaemic alkalosis*.

● *Loop diuretics*, for example frusemide 40–160 mg daily, bumetanide 1–4 mg daily and ethacrynic acid 50–100 mg daily.

Loop diuretics act mainly by inhibiting the reabsorption of chloride ions in the ascending loop of Henle.

● *Potassium sparing diuretics*, for example spironolactone 25–200 mg daily, amiloride 5–20 mg daily, triamterene 50–200 mg daily.

Potassium sparing diuretics act by inhibiting the resorption of sodium from the distal tubule. As a consequence reduced amounts of potassium and hydrogen are exchanged for sodium in this part of the tubule. In the presence of impaired renal function this can result in a metabolic acidosis and hyperkalaemia that occasionally may be dangerous.

Spironolactone is a true aldosterone antagonist and is inactive in adrenalectomised persons.

Side effects of the diuretics

● *Dehydration* that may lead to hypovolaemia and postural hypotension.
● *Electrolyte imbalance*
a   *The thiazide and loop diuretics* may cause hypokalaemic alkalosis.
b   *The potassium sparing diuretics* may cause hyperkalaemia and a metabolic acidosis.

c   *Hyponatraemia* may occasionally result from the increased excretion of sodium caused by diuretics.
● *Metabolic effects*
a   *Hyperuricaemia.* Thiazides and loop diuretics commonly cause hyperuricaemia and may occasionally precipitate clinical gout.
b   *Carbohydrate intolerance.* Thiazides and less commonly loop diuretics may worsen or precipitate diabetes.
c   *Lipids.* Thiazides cause a slight elevation of the plasma lipids.
d   *Endocrine disorders.* Spironolactone antagonises androgen activity and may cause gynaecomastia and impotence in males. Treatment of hypertension with thiazides has been shown to double the incidence of impotence in middle-aged men.

Digitalis: actions and side effects
Questions

27   How is digitalis thought to act at the enzyme/molecular level?
28i   What are the main therapeutic actions of digitalis on the failing left ventricle?
  ii   At what sites in the heart does digitalis act? What are its main actions in terms of heart rate, refractory period and speed of conduction at these sites?
29   What are the main side effects of digitalis?

Answers

27   Action of digitalis at the enzyme/molecular level

It is thought that digitalis achieves its positive inotropic action by inhibiting the enzyme $Na^+ - K^+$ ATPase in the wall of the cardiac muscle fibres. Normally this enzyme pumps sodium out of the cell. Under the influence of digitalis sodium therefore enters the cell. Through a separate sodium/calcium exchange mechanism the sodium that enters the cell is then exchanged for extracellular calcium. As a result intracellular calcium is increased and increases the contractility of the cardiac muscle fibres.

28i   The main therapeutic actions of digitalis on the failing left ventricle

● Increase in the strength of contraction (positive inotropic effect). Digitalis also increases the strength of contraction of the non-failing heart, but since this effect is only helpful in the failing heart, it is only with cardiac failure that the drug causes an increase of cardiac output.
● In patients with fast atrial fibrillation digitalis' main effect is to slow the ventricular rate of response to the fibrillating atria by inducing a degree of atrioventricular block. This increases cardiac efficiency as there is then more time for the ventricles to fill between beats.

28ii   The sites of action of digitalis and its effects at each site

These may be summarised as follows:
● *S-A node*. Although digitalis increases the power of contraction of the non-failing heart, its effect upon the *speed* of sinus rhythm in healthy persons is usually negligible. By contrast, in patients with *sinus rhythm and heart failure it slows the node*, mainly by a vagal effect, although at higher concentrations it also slows the node by a direct effect.
● *A-V node*. Digitalis slows conduction through and lengthens the refractory period of the A-V node in the same way as it affects the S-A node, that is mainly by a vagal effect although at higher concentrations it has a direct effect. In atrial fibrillation these effects block most of the numerous impulses passing down from the atria.
● *Purkinje conducting tissue*. Here the effect of digitalis is mainly a direct one causing:
a   slowing of conduction which may result in prolongation of the PR interval, and
b   lengthening of the refractory period.
● *Cardiac muscle*. The actions of digitalis here are opposite to those in the A-V node and Purkinje conducting tissue, and are a *direct effect* causing:
a   speeding of conduction, and
b   shortening of the refractory period of both atrial and ventricular muscle.

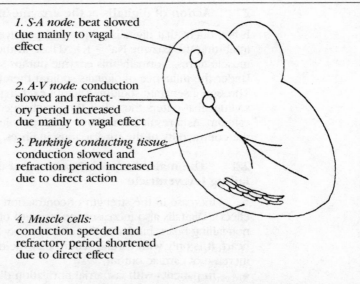

1. S-A node: beat slowed due mainly to vagal effect

2. A-V node: conduction slowed and refract-ory period increased due mainly to vagal effect

3. Purkinje conducting tissue: conduction slowed and refraction period increased due to direct action

4. Muscle cells: conduction speeded and refractory period shortened due to direct effect

Figure 15. Summary of the sites and actions of digitalis upon the failing heart

29   The main side effects of digitalis

Digitalis may cause almost any arrhythmia:

●   *Tachyarrhythmias.* These are due to the drug increasing the excitability of heart muscle by increasing the speed of conduction and reducing the refractory period of the muscle fibres. *Hypokalaemia potentiates this effect* due at least in part to the fact that the drug competes with potassium for binding sites on the enzyme $Na^+ - K^+$ ATPase. In the presence of hypokalaemia increased amounts of the drug are bound to the enzyme and so potentiate the drug's side effects. Ventricular and junctional arrhythmias are more commonly caused by digitalis than supraventricular arrhythmias. In ascending order of frequency and seriousness these ventricular arrhythmias are:

a   Ventricular extrasystoles.
b   Pulsus bigeminus (coupling).
c   Ventricular tachycardia.
d   Ventricular fibrillation.

Less commonly digitalis may cause *junctional and supraventricular arrhythmias* such as:

a   Atrial extrasystoles.
b   Paroxysmal supraventricular tachycardia.
c   Atrial fibrillation often with a very slow ventricular rate due to the increased refractory period of the A-V node.

●   *Bradyarrhythmias.* These are due to slowing of the S-A node and to slowing of conduction along the bundle and to the increased refractory period of the A-V node. The bradyarrhythmias caused by digitalis are:

a   Sinus bradycardia.
b   Heart block of any degree, including occasionally third degree heart block.

●   *Gastrointestinal upsets:*

a   Anorexia, nausea and vomiting due to stimulation of the vomiting centre in the brain stem. In chronic digitalis toxicity this may contribute to cardiac cachexia.
b   Diarrhoea.

●   *Visual changes* including blurring of vision, or yellow vision known as cinchonism.

●   *Nervous system changes* including fatigue and restlessness.

●   *Gynaecomastia.*

Comment

The potential seriousness of the side effects of digitalis are well illustrated by the following case. A 63 year old man, Mr S-M, was admitted to a coronary care unit with an acute full thickness anterior myocardial infarct. About 12 hours after admission he developed atrial fibrillation for which he was treated with digoxin 0.25 mg 6 hourly. The doctor making the prescription intended to adjust the dose the following day and so no stop date was put on the prescription. Unfortunately the doctor was taken ill and the other members of the medical team failed to check the prescription chart properly. Five days later the patient developed intractable ventricular fibrillation from which he died despite all efforts at resuscitation.

This case illustrates two important points, firstly that overdosage with digoxin may be lethal, secondly that *it is essential to carefully check every prescription a patient is receiving each time he or she is seen.*

Digitalis in clinical practice
Questions

30   What are the three main clinical indications for administering digitalis?

31i   What are the two most commonly used preparations of digitalis? What are their usual doses? What is the main mode of excretion of each? What are their usual half lives?

  ii   What are the indications for measuring plasma digitalis levels?

  iii   List the factors likely to increase a patient's sensitivity to and side effects from digitalis.

32   What other commonly used drugs cause elevation of the serum level of digoxin?

33i   After what amount of *digoxin* administered orally are most patients digitalised? Suggest a dosage schedule for oral digitalisation.

  ii   How would you urgently digitalise a patient?

Answers

30   The three main clinical indications for the administration of digitalis

These follow from its therapeutic and electrical actions outlined in the answer to question 28. They are:

●   *To slow the rate and increase the efficiency of the ventricles in atrial fibrillation.* Except for a few patients who have a spontaneously slow ventricular rate, to avoid an excessively high ventricular rate during exercise all patients with atrial fibrillation should be digitalised.

Digitalis is also sometimes used in the acute treatment of both paroxysmal supraventricular tachycardia and atrial flutter, although verapamil 5–10 mg intravenously is probably the drug of choice in this situation. If used, digitalis probably achieves its effect in paroxysmal supraventricular tachycardia by its vagal effect. In atrial flutter it slows the ventricular response by inducing a degree of A-V block. In addition, because of its direct effects on atrial muscle it tends to convert atrial flutter to atrial fibrillation which occasionally reverts to sinus rhythm if the drug is stopped.

●   *Cardiac failure*

a   *With atrial fibrillation.* The reasons for this are explained in the first part of the answer to question 28.

b   *With sinus rhythm*. The main beneficial effect of digitalis in
this situation is due to its positive inotropic effect. With the advent
of modern diuretics the need for this has become relatively less
important than previously, and so in patients with cardiac failure
and sinus rhythm digitalis is now usually reserved for those
patients whose condition is not adequately controlled by diuretics
alone or diuretics plus vasodilators. For this reason most patients
with well controlled cardiac failure and sinus rhythm *do not* need
maintenance digitalis.
●   *Prevention of recurrent paroxysmal supraventricular
arrhythmias* such as paroxysmal atrial fibrillation or paroxysmal
supraventricular tachycardia.
     Alternative drugs used in this situation include quinidine,
disopyramide, flecainide and amiodarone.

31i   The two most commonly used preparations of digitalis

●   Digoxin
●   Digitoxin

	Digoxin	*Digitoxin*
Usual daily maintenance dose	0.125 mg daily to 0.25 mg three times a day	0.1–0.2 mg
Mode of excretion	85% renal	85% hepatic
Usual half life	1.6 days	5 days
Protein binding	20%	90%

Digoxin is more commonly prescribed than digitoxin. The main
indication for digitoxin is the presence of renal impairment. In
uraemia the half lives of the two preparations are: digoxin about
4½ days, digitoxin about 7 days.

31ii   Indications for measuring plasma digitalis levels

Plasma levels of digitalis do not need to be measured routinely.
The main indications for measuring plasma levels of the drug are:
●   Suspected toxicity.
●   Renal impairment with a high blood urea.
●   Patients requiring an unusually high maintenance dose.

The accepted therapeutic plasma level of digoxin is 1–2 ng/l. For
digitoxin the accepted level is 10–15 times as much due to
protein binding.

31iii   The factors likely to increase a patient's sensitivity to and side effects from digitalis

●   *Advanced age*. Often in part due to decreased renal
clearance of the drug.
●   *Advanced ventricular disease*.

- *Renal impairment.* Especially with digoxin.
- *Electrolyte upset*

Hypokalaemia
Hypomagnesaemia   Most commonly caused by
Hyponatraemia   diuretic therapy
Hypercalcaemia

- *Hypothyroidism.* The half life of the drug is prolonged in this condition.
- *Hypoxia.* For example cor pulmonale.
- *The sick sinus syndrome or disease of the A-V node.*

32   Elevation of serum digitalis levels by other drugs

Serum levels of digitalis may be elevated by decreased renal clearance caused by the concomitant administration of:
- Verapamil
- Amiodarone—which also competes with digitalis for protein binding
- Nifedipine
- Quinidine

33i   Oral digitalisation with digoxin

In theory a patient is digitalised when their body stores of the drug are in a steady state and are sufficient to have the desired therapeutic effect. In practice the digitalising or loading dose of digoxin is 1-2 mg. Orally this is usually given in divided doses whose size and frequency is determined by the speed with which a therapeutic effect is desired. Depending upon the clinical situation, typical schedules are:
- 1 mg immediately followed by 0.25 mg 6-8 hourly for 3-4 doses
- 0.5 mg 6-8 hourly for 3-4 doses
- 0.25 mg 6-8 hourly for 4-6 doses

33ii   Urgent digitalisation

The main indication for this is intractable life threatening acute left ventricular failure. In this situation urgent digitalisation may be achieved by the intravenous administration over half to one hour of 200 ml 5% dextrose containing either digoxin 0.5-1.0 mg or ouabain 1 mg.

Drugs that reduce the work of the heart by reducing preload and afterload (the vasodilators)

Question

34   List the main drugs that act this way. What is the main pharmacological action of each of them?

Answer

34   The main vasodilators

These drugs may be divided into (a) those whose main action is to cause relaxation of *arterial* vascular smooth muscle, and (b) those whose main action is to cause relaxation of vascular smooth muscle in the capacitance vessels or *veins*.

Arterial dilators

These drugs cause a decrease in peripheral resistance and as a consequence lower afterload and tend to cause an increase in cardiac output. They are therefore particularly useful in the relief of symptoms due to low cardiac output such as fatigue.

Drug	Mode of action
● Captopril 6.25–50 mg three times daily	Inhibitor of the enzyme converting angiotension I to the powerful vasoconstrictor, angiotension II
● Enalapril 2.5–20 mg daily	
● Hydrallazine 25 mg three times daily to 50 mg four times daily	Direct relaxation of vascular smooth muscle
● Nifedipine 5–20 mg three times daily	Calcium channel blocker
● Prazosin 1 mg three times daily to 5 mg four times daily	Competitive inhibition of post-synaptic alpha$_1$ adrenoreceptors

Venous dilators

These drugs cause relaxation of vascular smooth muscle in the walls of veins. As a result blood is redistributed away from the congested great central veins to the capacitance veins, particularly of the muscles and gut. This causes lowering of preload, and in particular relief of symptoms due to congestion such as dyspnoea.

Drug	Mode of action
● Morphine 5–10 mg intravenously Diamorphine 5 mg intravenously	Direct relaxation of vascular smooth muscle
● Nitrates: various oral, buccal and intravenous preparations	Direct relaxation of vascular smooth muscle

Heart transplantation
Question

35 What are the indications for heart transplantation?

Answer

35 Indications

Heart transplantation is a treatment option for patients aged up to 60-65 years who are invalided with intractable cardiac failure despite full treatment along the lines suggested on page 43, provided there is no irreversible pulmonary hypertension or damage to other organs causing conditions such as renal failure, and no readily correctable surgical lesion such as valvular stenosis or incompetence or a resectable cardiac aneurysm.

Further Reading

Braunwald E (ed) (1984). *Heart Disease*, 2nd edition. WB Saunders, Philadelphia. Chapters 9, cardiac catheterization; 15, clinical manifestations; 16, management of heart failure; 39, cardiomyopathies.

Weatherall DJ, Ledingham JGG, Warrell DA (eds) (1987). *Oxford Textbook of Medicine*, 2nd edition. Oxford University Press, Oxford. The cardiomyopathies, pp 13.209-29.

Case B   **A Case of Palpitations: Mr J-W, aged 65 years**

A happily married retired builder's clerk who smoked 15 cigarettes per day and was admitted to hospital with a one hour history of rapid heart beat and feelings of breathlessness and dizziness.

On examination he presented as a gaunt middle-aged man with a lined smoker's face. Otherwise clinical examination was normal except for a rapid regular pulse 170 beats per minute and blood pressure 95/70. Electrocardiograph showed changes compatible with paroxysmal supraventricular tachycardia (PSVT). With appropriate treatment along the lines suggested later in Chapter 3 he was restored to sinus rhythm, and on the following day was discharged home.

Chapter 3
Bradyarrhythmias, Bundle Branch Block, Tachyarrhythmias

The bradyarrhythmias
Questions

1   List the causes of sinus bradycardia.

2   What is the sick sinus syndrome? What are its causes? By what four patterns does it manifest itself? What are its clinical effects? How is it treated?

3i   Describe the three degrees of heart block. What are Mobitz types I + II heart block?

ii   List the causes of heart block.

iii   How might the various degrees of heart block present clinically? How is heart block treated?

iv   Describe a Stokes–Adams attack.

Answers

1   The causes of sinus bradycardia

By convention sinus bradycardia is said to be present when there is sinus rhythm at a rate less than 60 beats per minute. It may be caused by:

Vagotonia

● Physiological, for example in highly trained athletes.
● A faint or vasovagal attack.
● Massage of the carotid sinus, eyeball compression, or the Valsalva manoeuvre in which the subject voluntarily increases his or her intrathoracic pressure by expiring against a closed glottis.
● Raised intracranial pressure.

Drugs

● Digitalis, due mainly to vagotonia, although at high concentrations direct depression of the S-A node also occurs.
● Beta blocking drugs reducing sympathetic drive to the heart.
● Neostigmine, due to a vagotonic/cholinergic effect.

Miscellaneous conditions

- Myocardial infarction due either to vagotonia reversible with atropine, or to ischaemic dysfunction of the S-A node.
- Severe jaundice.
- Hypothyroidism.
- The sick sinus syndrome.
- Hypothermia.

2   The sick sinus syndrome

This is a condition associated with dysfunction of the S-A node and its pacemaker activity. Usually it is due to degenerate fibrosis, although it may also be caused by ischaemia, drugs such as digitalis and quinidine, infiltration with amyloid or tumour, or a cardiomyopathy. Four patterns of sick sinus syndrome are recognised:

- *Sinus bradycardia*—sinus rhythm at an unexplained rate of less than 50–60 beats per minute.
- *Alternating periods of bradycardia and tachycardia* (the tachy–brady syndrome).
- *Sinoatrial block* in which the sinus node impulse fails to cross into the atrium. This is an intermittent phenomenon and results in sudden complete loss of a P wave and the following QRS complex and a gap in otherwise regular sinus rhythm. It has to be differentiated from Mobitz type II heart block in which a P wave occurs without a following QRS complex (see page 57).
- *Sinus arrest* in which there is no activity of the S-A node. This results in a slow pulse without any P waves on the ECG. It is therefore different from complete heart block in which there is atrioventricular disassociation with P waves independent of the QRS complexes. If the atrium is electrically unstable it may lead to atrial fibrillation.

Clinically the sick sinus syndrome is manifested by palpitations, dizziness and syncope. Drug treatment may make it worse. In symptomatic persons cardiac pacing is indicated.

3   Heart block

i   Heart block is associated with delay or obstruction in conduction of the electrical impulse from the atria to the ventricles.

- *First degree heart block* is usually due to delay at the A-V node and results in sinus rhythm with a PR interval greater than 0.2 seconds. In young people first degree heart block may be due to vagotonia.
- *Second degree heart block* is associated with complete failure of some or many supraventricular impulses reaching the ventricles. In the *Wenckebach phenomenon or Mobitz type I heart block* the degree of A-V block gradually increases over a sequence of beats. This results in gradual lengthening of the PR interval over

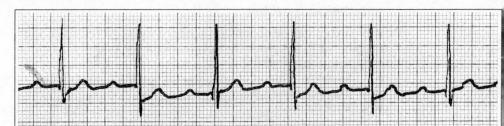

Figure 16. *First degree heart block* showing prolonged PR interval > 0.2 seconds (> one big square or five small squares on the ECG paper).

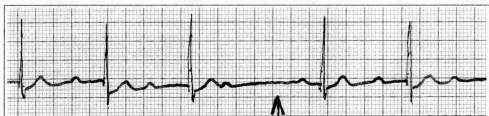

Figure 17. *Mobitz Type I heart block (Wenkebach phenomenon)* showing gradual prolongation of the PR interval over three beats followed by failure of conduction of the fourth beat and loss of QRS complexes indicated by arrows.

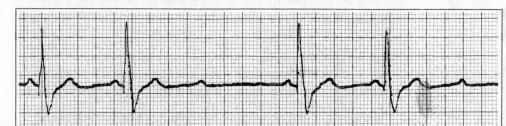

Figure 18. *Mobitz Type II heart block* showing intermittent phenomenon of a P wave without a following QRS complex.

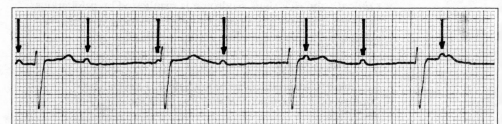

Figure 19. Complete heart block showing complete dissociation between the atria and ventricles. The p waves are marked by arrows.

three or four beats until a point is reached at which the A-V block is sufficient to completely obstruct the conduction of the next atrial beat across the node. This results in failure to initiate a ventricular beat, and on the ECG a P wave without a following QRS complex. In the pulse there is a gap of one beat. Typically, the A-V node then recovers and the process repeats itself.

In Mobitz type II heart block the PR interval is constant but there is intermittent failure of conduction of the atrial impulse to the ventricles. A P wave therefore occurs without a following QRS complex. This may affect a single beat or multiple beats. If it is multiple there will be marked gaps in the pulse and syncope may occur.

• *Third degree heart block* is associated with total failure of conduction of the atrial impulse to the ventricles. The atria and the ventricles therefore beat regularly but at different rates, the ventricular rate depending upon the site of the pacemaker within it. Usually the ventricular rate is 30-40 beats per minute.

ii   *Causes of heart block* are:
• Myocardial infarction
• Digitalis toxicity
• Idiopathic fibrosis—the commonest cause in the elderly
• Aortic valve disease—especially aortic stenosis
• Rheumatic fever
• Congenital
• Cardiac surgery
• Inflammatory processes such as sarcoidosis or the collagenoses

iii   *Clinical features of heart block:* First degree and Mobitz type I heart block do not cause symptoms, but may progress to complete heart block. Mobitz type II heart block with multiple pulse gaps and third degree heart block may be asymptomatic or cause dizziness, syncope or heart failure. Because pacing considerably prolongs the life of those with complete heart block, whether or not it is causing symptoms complete heart block should be treated with a pacemaker, as should symptomatic second degree heart block. First degree and symptomless second degree heart block do not require a pacemaker. Temporary pacing after myocardial infarction is discussed on page 128.

iv   *A Stokes-Adams attack* is an abrupt loss of consciousness due to transient ventricular standstill caused for instance by Mobitz type II or third degree heart block, or transient ventricular fibrillation. The patient falls unconscious, and is pulseless and pale. After an interval of up to one or two minutes recovery occurs. Unlike epilepsy, recovery is usually sudden, and may be accompanied by flushing of the skin as the circulation starts up again. However, it is important to appreciate that due to cerebral anoxia a Stokes-Adams attack may cause a full blown epileptic seizure.

Bundle branch block and axis deviation
Question

4i   What is bundle branch block?
 ii   What is the significance of left bundle branch block, and of right bundle branch block?

iii   What are the signs of left bundle branch block, and of right bundle branch block?

iv   What are the ECG changes associated with left bundle branch block and with right bundle branch block? How may they be explained?

v   Describe left axis deviation, and right axis deviation.

vi   What is left anterior hemi-block, and what is left posterior hemi-block?

Answer

4   Bundle branch block

i   Bundle branch block is due to conduction of the electrical impulse along only one or two of the three fascicles of the bundle of His beneath the A-V node.

ii   *The significance of bundle branch block.* Left bundle branch block always signifies disease of the conducting tissue. Isolated right bundle branch block may signify disease but may also occur in normals. Particularly after myocardial infarction, the development of bundle branch block may be a harbinger of complete heart block with all its attendant problems.

iii   *Signs.* On its own bundle branch block is associated with sinus rhythm and does not produce symptoms. The signs are mainly those of any underlying heart disease. In addition, as explained on page 18, with left bundle branch block closure of the aortic valve is delayed, leading to narrowing of the split of the second heart sound during inspiration, whereas normally, of course, the split widens with inspiration. With right bundle branch block the first heart sound is widely split due to delayed closure of the tricuspid valve.

iv   *ECG changes.* Bundle branch block is associated with wide complexes, > 0.12 seconds duration. The reason for this is that although depolarisation of each ventricle is of normal duration, depolarisation of the two sides does not occur simultaneously, but is delayed to one side or the other. To understand bundle branch block it is necessary to appreciate that normally depolarisation in the ventricles starts in the septum and travels across the septum from left to right producing the first small wave of the QRS complex.

In *left bundle branch block* conduction to the left side of the septum is blocked. Conduction within the septum therefore occurs in a reversed manner from the right bundle to the left. The sequence of events this triggers is illustrated in Figure 20. In the lateral leads, V4-6, I and aVl, depolarisation of the *septum* from right to left produces the first of the two R waves as the impulse travels towards the recording electrode. Normal conduction to the right ventricle, away from the electrode, then produces an S wave that is followed by the second R wave as the delayed impulse is conducted to the left ventricle. As illustrated, in lead V1 over the right ventricle, the waves produced are in the opposite direction. Because the left ventricle dominates the pattern of electrical events in all leads, the electrocardiograph shows wide complexes throughout.

Right bundle branch block is seen best in lead V_1. Normal conduction from left to right in the septum produces the first small R wave as the impulse travels towards the recording electrode. Normal conduction to the left ventricle, away from lead V_1, then produces the normal S or down wave seen in this lead. Delayed conduction to the blocked right ventricle then produces the second R wave. The result is a wide complex known as rSR[1]. In the lateral leads, V_{4-6}, I and aVl the delayed conduction to the right ventricle, away from the recording electrode, produces a wide S wave.

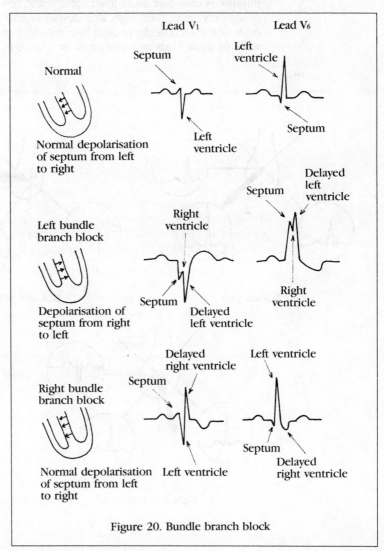

Figure 20. Bundle branch block

v   *Axis deviation.* Normally the main component of the electrical impulse is towards ECG lead II. The term axis deviation refers to deviation from this. With left axis deviation (LAD) the axis is swung anti-clockwise or horizontally as a result of left anterior hemi-block, left ventricular hypertrophy or conditions that lift the heart such as abdominal obesity and ascites. With right axis deviation (RAD) the axis is swung clockwise or vertically by conditions such as left posterior hemi-block, right ventricular hypertrophy, and emphysema causing the heart to hang vertically in the chest.

As Figure 21 shows, axis deviation is associated with movement of the electrically neutral line. With left axis deviation leads III and aVf are behind the line. The direction of the electrical impulse is therefore away from these leads, resulting in a negative, down or S wave. With right axis deviation leads III and aVf are in front of the electrically neutral line, resulting in a positive or R wave in these leads and a negative or S wave in leads I and aVl.

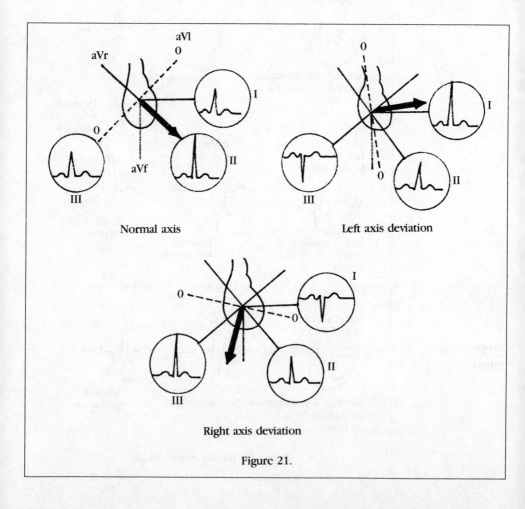

Normal axis

Left axis deviation

Right axis deviation

Figure 21.

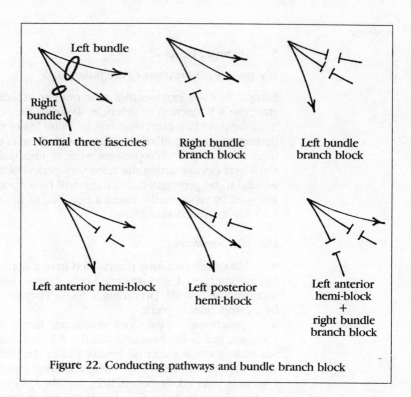

Figure 22. Conducting pathways and bundle branch block

vi   *Left anterior hemi-block and left posterior hemi-block.* As their names imply, and as is illustrated in Figure 22, these conditions are associated with block of one of the two fascicles to the left ventricle, namely the anterior and the posterior fascicles respectively. On the ECG they are associated with normal or slightly wide QRS complexes. Left anterior hemi-block is also associated with left axis deviation, and left posterior hemi-block with right axis deviation.

Left anterior hemi-block is important after myocardial infarction, because when combined with right bundle branch block it carries the implication that two of the three fascicles have been affected by the infarct and that complete heart block will occur if the infarct extends to involve the third fascicle.

Ectopic beats or extrasystoles
Question

5   Describe both the rhythm and quality of the pulse in a patient with ectopic beats or extrasystoles.

Describe the ECG abnormalities of an atrial ectopic beat, a junctional ectopic beat, a ventricular ectopic beat.

What is the significance of ventricular ectopic beats?

Answer

5   Ectopic beats

The quality and rhythm of the pulse

Ectopic beats or extrasystoles arise from an ectopic focus in the atria, the A-V junction or ventricle. Typically they cause irregularities of an otherwise regular pulse. As ectopics are premature, cardiac filling associated with them is usually incomplete and the ectopic beat weak or impalpable. If the next sinus beat occurs during the refractory period of an ectopic beat it will fail to be propagated and there will be a compensatory pause followed by an unusually forceful beat due to the extra time available for ventricular filling.

ECG abnormalities

● *Atrial ectopics* look normal and have a normal QRS complex, but are interposed, and preceded by a P wave that is early or even superimposed on the preceding T wave. They are usually followed by a compensatory pause.
● *Junctional ectopics* look similar and have a normal QRS complex, but as the beat arises in the A-V junction rather than the S-A node, there is either no P wave before the QRS complex, or if atrial contraction occurs by retrograde firing into the atrium, the P wave is inverted, or occurs late, after the QRS complex.
    Junctional tachycardia consists of runs of these beats.
● *Ventricular ectopics* appear as large wide 'ugly' complexes among the normal supraventricular beats. They are of duration > 0.12 seconds. They are usually associated with a compensatory pause.

The significance of ventricular ectopic beats

In healthy people they are probably of no significance. In the presence of heart disease they may indicate an impaired prognosis.

Supraventricular tachyarrhythmias (i): classification, description and causes
Questions

6   Give a simple classification of the supraventricular tachycardias.
7   Give a pictorial description of what is happening in the heart, describe the electrical abnormalities thought to occur, and describe the ECG changes associated with: (a) paroxysmal supraventricular tachycardia, (b) atrial flutter, and (c) atrial fibrillation.
    Which is the commonest of these arrythmias? In which ECG leads is atrial flutter usually most easily seen?
8   List the generally accepted most common causes of the above supraventricular tachycardias.

Answers

6   A simple classification of the supraventricular tachycardias

The easiest way to understand the supraventricular tachycardias is to appreciate that for most clinical purposes they may be divided into three, and that these three are most conveniently classified by considering the speed of the atrial waves they produce. In ascending order of speed of the atrial waves they are:

Arrhythmia	*Speed of atrial waves (beats per minute)*
● Paroxysmal supraventricular tachycardia (PSVT)	160–230 approximately
● Atrial flutter	230–330 approximately
● Atrial fibrillation (AF)	400–500 (f or fibrillation waves)

7   Pictorial description, electrical abnormalities and ECG changes associated with the supraventricular tachycardias

● *Paroxysmal supraventricular tachycardia (PSVT)*. In about 20% of cases this arrhythmia is due to re-entry, which is described below, or an ectopic focus within the atrium. In about 40% of cases it is associated with the repeated circulation of an impulse within the A-V node, and in the remaining 40% of cases with a second or extra bundle of conducting tissue between the atria and ventricles that together with the Purkinje conducting tissue forms

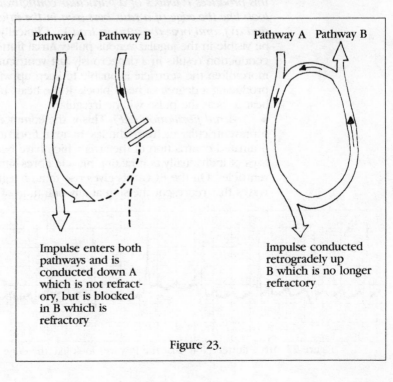

Pathway A   Pathway B   Pathway A Pathway B

Impulse enters both pathways and is conducted down A which is not refractory, but is blocked in B which is refractory

Impulse conducted retrogradely up B which is no longer refractory

Figure 23.

a circle that allows impulses to pass backwards and forwards between the atria and ventricles in a circular fashion.

The circulation of impulses within the atrium, the A-V node or via an extra bundle is known as *re-entry* and occurs in situations in which there are two conduction pathways with different refractory periods and different conduction velocities as shown in Figure 23.

The resulting arrhythmia is fast and *regular* with a rate of 160–230 beats per minute. Because the impulses come from the A-V node or atria *the ECG looks normal but very fast*, unless there is bundle branch block in which case the ECG is fast and regular with wide complexes. P waves may or may not be seen.

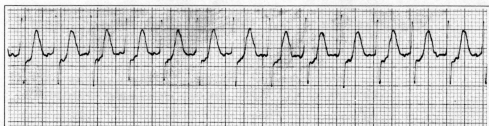

Figure 24. Paroxysmal Atrial Tachycardia. Note the fast rate, regularity and normal shape of the ventricular complexes.

- *Atrial flutter*. This arrhythmia is due to an ectopic focus, or to a circular wave going round the atrium causing atrial contractions at the rate of 230–330 beats per minute. *On the ECG this produces P waves of a particular configuration or shape that look like the edge of a saw, best seen in the inferior leads II, III and aVf, and over the atria in lead V_1.* Clinically, flutter waves may be visible in the jugular venous pulse. Atrial flutter with 1 : 1 conduction results in a dangerously fast ventricular rate, although more often the ventricle is unable to keep up with the atria, producing a degree of heart block. If the heart block varies from beat to beat the pulse will be irregular.

- *Atrial fibrillation (AF)*. This is the commonest of the supraventricular tachyarrythmias. In atrial fibrillation there is no co-ordinated contraction of the atria which have become shimmering bags of individually contracting muscle fibres sitting on top of the ventricles. On the ECG this gives rise to an irregular baseline of f waves that represent the sum at any one time of the action

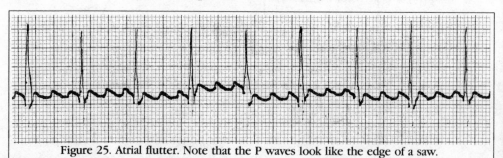

Figure 25. Atrial flutter. Note that the P waves look like the edge of a saw.

potentials produced by the haphazard contraction of dozens or hundreds of individually contracting atrial muscle fibres. Impulses pass haphazardly from the atria to the ventricles causing irregular ventricular contractions and an irregular pulse. Because the pulse is irregular the time available for ventricular filling varies causing a variable stroke volume. As a result in atrial fibrillation both the rate and the strength of the pulse vary continuously. Some beats are too weak to produce a perceptible peripheral pulse. The result is a deficit in the rate of the radial pulse compared with the apical pulse. Because of this the apex rate should always be used during clinical assessment of the heart rate in patients with atrial fibrillation.

On the ECG atrial fibrillation is characterised by an irregular baseline of f waves (and absence of proper P waves), and irregular ventricular complexes of a normal shape.

The irregular pulse caused by atrial fibrillation has to be differentiated from the other causes of an irregular pulse. This is discussed in the answer to question 18 on page 75.

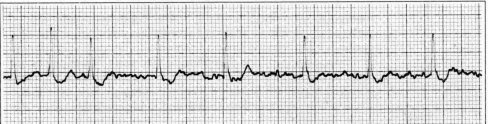

Figure 26. Atrial fibrillation. Note the irregular f waves of the base line and the r irregular rate of the ventricular complexes.

8 Causes of the supraventricular tachycardias

Paroxysmal supraventricular tachycardia generally occurs in persons with abnormal circuits or re-entry pathways without heart disease.

Atrial fibrillation and atrial flutter may be caused by conditions that irritate or excite the atria, thus:

● Myocardial infarction and ischaemic heart disease.
● Hypertensive heart disease.
● Thyrotoxicosis.
● Mitral valve disease (mitral stenosis and mitral regurgitation) as a result of the big baggy left atrium found in these conditions becoming electrically unstable.
● Infection, particularly of the respiratory tract.
● Cardiomyopathy.
● Tumours, for instance carcinoma of the bronchus involving the pericardium.
● Pulmonary embolus.
● Alcoholic binge.
● Drugs. Due to the fact that it increases the excitability of heart muscle, digitalis may induce arrhythmias. Most commonly these are ventricular; occasionally they are supraventricular.

Supraventricular tachyarrhythmias (ii): cardioversion and anticoagulation in atrial fibrillation; the Wolff–Parkinson–White syndrome

Questions

9   In which group of patients is it usual to accept atrial fibrillation, and in which fibrillating patients is it usual to attempt restoration of sinus rhythm?

10   To which organs are arterial emboli from a fibrillating left atrium likely to disseminate? What is their likely effect on those organs? What are the indications for long-term anticoagulation in patients with chronic atrial fibrillation?

11   Describe the Wolff–Parkinson–White syndrome. Explain the ECG abnormalities associated with it. With which arrhythmias is it associated?

Answers

9   Atrial fibrillation: acceptance versus conversion to sinus rhythm

● *Paroxysmal supraventricular tachycardia and atrial flutter.* Because they eventually result in cardiac failure persistent paroxysmal supraventricular tachycardia and atrial flutter should generally be converted to sinus rhythm.

● *Acceptance of atrial fibrillation.* Because of its tendency to recur in the middle-aged and elderly, in persons aged over about 60, atrial fibrillation is usually accepted although patients with it are generally given digitalis to prevent an unacceptably fast ventricular rate.

● *Conversion of atrial fibrillation to sinus rhythm.* In younger persons, especially those in whom no obvious cause for atrial fibrillation is apparent, a condition known as 'lone atrial fibrillation', and in those who have had a mitral valvotomy or treatment of thyrotoxicosis, most authorities advise action to restore *persistent* atrial fibrillation to sinus rhythm.

10   Embolisation from a fibrillating left atrium, and the indications for long-term anticoagulation in chronic atrial fibrillation

Because the atria do not contract or empty normally in patients with atrial fibrillation, stasis occurs that may lead to thrombus formation, particularly in the atrial appendage. As a consequence there is a risk of systemic arterial emboli from the fibrillating left atrium, and occasionally of pulmonary emboli from the fibrillating right atrium. The most common sites of systemic embolisation are:

Site	Effect
● Brain	Stroke or transient ischaemic attack
● Leg	Ischaemia or gangrene
● Kidney	Infarction
● Superior mesenteric artery	Ischaemia or infarction of small bowel
● Coronary artery	Angina or myocardial infarction
● Spleen	Infarction

Atrial fibrillation combined with mitral stenosis

Due to the increased stasis produced in the left atrium by the combination of atrial fibrillation and the large baggy left atrium associated with mitral stenosis the risk of arterial embolisation is particularly great in this situation. Trials have shown that the benefits of long-term anticoagulation, for instance with warfarin, far outweigh the risks of haemorrhage. Unless contraindicated, all patients with atrial fibrillation and mitral stenosis should therefore be anticoagulated.

Atrial fibrillation combined with mitral regurgitation

In this situation long-term anticoagulation is indicated in those cases in which *severe* mitral regurgitation has resulted in the left atrium enlarging to more than about 4 cm diameter. With lesser forms of mitral regurgitation and atrial fibrillation anticoagulants are usually reserved for the indications suggested in the next paragraph.

Atrial fibrillation without mitral valve disease

Although there is still a benefit from long-term anticoagulation, in this situation it is less strong than with mitral stenosis, and as a consequence persons in this category are usually not anticoagulated, although some authorities advise anticoagulation if the left atrium is large, for instance greater than 4 cm diameter on echocardiogram. In addition, except when contraindicated, it is undoubtedly wise to anticoagulate any person with atrial fibrillation in whom there is a suspicion of arterial emboli, although in the case of suspected cerebral emboli a computerised tomographic (CT) brain scan should be performed first to exclude cerebral haemorrhage as anticoagulants are contraindicated by the presence of haemorrhage.

11   The Wolff–Parkinson–White syndrome

This is a congenital disorder due to an accessory or extra conducting pathway between the atria and the ventricles known as a bundle of Kent. This pathway allows electrical impulses to bypass the A-V node and its delaying effect upon conduction. As a result conduction between the atria and ventricles is abnormally fast. Because the abnormal delta wave occurs before the R wave, the PR interval *appears* to be short, although in fact the interval from the top of the P wave to the top of the R wave is normal. The delta wave is due to the abnormally fast spread of the impulse through the ventricle from the accessory pathway, and the normal R wave to spread of the impulse from the normal conducting tissue.

The WPW syndrome, as it is known, is associated with paroxysms of atrial fibrillation and a re-entrant form of paroxysmal supraventricular tachycardia of the type described on page 63. Because of fast conduction between the atria and the ventricles, the ventricular rate may be dangerously fast with the atrial fibrillation associated with the WPW syndrome.

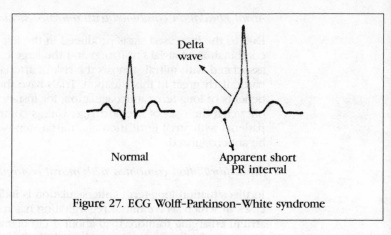

Figure 27. ECG Wolff-Parkinson-White syndrome

Supraventricular tachyarrhythmias (iii): treatment
Questions

12 List the various types of therapy available for the treatment of the supraventricular tachycardias.

13 What are the indications for DC shock in the supraventricular tachycardias? How much power is usually required? What is the potential danger of shocking a digitalised patient?

14 The Vaughan Williams classification divides the anti-arrhythmic drugs into four classes. Describe the four classes, and the electrical and physiological phenomena upon which they are based, and give examples of drugs belonging to each class.

15 Write short notes on the following drugs used in the treatment of the supraventricular tachycardias. Which arrhythmias are they used for, what are their modes of action, dosage and main side effects:

i   Digitalis.
ii   Beta blocking drugs.
iii Verapamil.
iv   Quinidine, disopyramide and flecainide.
v   Amiodarone.

Answers

12 The various types of therapy available for the treatment of the supraventricular tachycardias

● *Mechanical procedures* such as massage of the carotid sinus, eyeball compression or the Valsalva manoeuvre. These procedures cause an increase of vagal tone. *The most efficient is the Valsalva manoeuvre* performed in the supine position by getting the patient to expire forcefully against a closed glottis. Using this method up to 20% of cases of paroxysmal supraventricular tachycardia may be converted to sinus rhythm. With atrial flutter the ventricular rate may slow temporarily whilst the procedure is applied; with atrial fibrillation there is usually no effect.

- *Drugs*. Digitalis remains the drug of choice for treating atrial fibrillation. Intravenous verapamil is the drug most commonly used for the conversion of paroxysmal supraventricular tachycardia and atrial flutter to sinus rhythm. Otherwise, choice is largely a matter of experience and monitoring response. The individual drugs most commonly prescribed are discussed below.
- *Direct current (DC) shock*. This acts by depolarising the myocardial cells and allowing the normal impulse to take over control of the heart beat.

13   Direct current shock and the supraventricular tachycardias

Indications

- Failure of response to drug therapy.
- Patients who are acutely ill with an arrhythmia and cardiac failure or hypotension. In this situation DC shock is often the anti-arrhythmic treatment of first choice, partly for reasons of speed, but also because many anti-arrhythmic drugs have negative inotropic effects, that is decrease the force of contraction of the cardiac muscle.

The power required

The amount of energy required to convert a supraventricular tachycardia is usually between 25 and 100 joules (up to 200 joules is often needed for ventricular tachyarrhythmias).

The potential danger of shocking a digitalised patient

As discussed on page 47, digitalis increases the excitability of heart muscle. In patients who are digitalised there is therefore a slight risk of DC shock causing ventricular fibrillation, although this is less likely now that defibrillators may be synchronised to deliver the shock on the R wave at the time of ventricular depolarisation. Nonetheless, if possible digitalis should be omitted for one or two days before cardioversion, particularly if there is any suspicion of drug toxicity.

Digitalis competes with potassium for binding sites on heart muscle. As a result hypokalaemia is associated with increased binding of digitalis to the heart, and as a consequence an increased danger of DC shock causing ventricular fibrillation.

14   The Vaughan Williams classification of anti-arrhythmic drugs

To a great extent this has been derived from the in-vitro effect of various drugs upon the action potential of normal cardiac muscle. Its main disadvantage is that it does not accommodate digitalis.

The rapid phase of depolarisation is caused by the fast entry of sodium ions into the myocardial cells. The plateau of the action potential is maintained by the slow entry of calcium ions into the

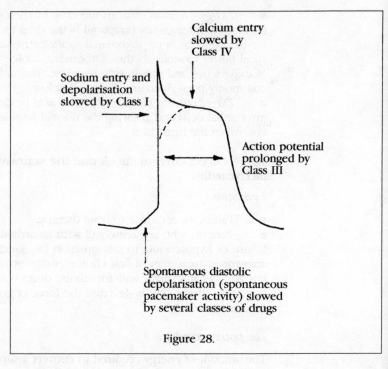

Calcium entry
slowed by
Class IV

Sodium entry and
depolarisation
slowed by Class I

Action potential
prolonged by
Class III

Spontaneous diastolic
depolarisation (spontaneous
pacemaker activity) slowed
by several classes of drugs

Figure 28.

cell. With this in mind the actions of the drugs in classes I, III and IV may be summarised as shown in Figure 28.

Class I

These drugs cause slowing of the fast entry of sodium ions into the cell and reduce the maximum rate of depolarisation. They are subdivided into:

Class Ia: In addition these drugs lengthen the duration of the action potential.
● Quinidine
● Disopyramide
● Procainamide (no longer used)

Class Ib: In addition these drugs shorten the duration of the action potential, and are effective only against ventricular arrhythmias.
● Lignocaine
● Mexiletine

Class Ic: These drugs have no effect upon the duration of the action potential.
● Flecainide
● Encainide (an experimental drug)

Class II

These drugs diminish the effects upon the heart of the catecholamines.
● Beta blockers
● Bretylium

Class III

These drugs prolong the duration of the action potential and hence the effective refractory period without altering the rate of depolarisation.

- Sotalol
- Amiodarone

Class IV

These drugs are the calcium antagonists, and slow the influx of calcium ions into the cell thereby maintaining the plateau of the action potential.

- Verapamil
- Diltiazem
- Tiapamil

15   Drugs used in treatment of supraventricular tachycardias

i   *Digitalis* is the drug of choice for the treatment of atrial fibrillation, although it is also used for the treatment of paroxysmal supraventricular tachycardia, and atrial flutter which it sometimes converts to either sinus rhythm or atrial fibrillation. It is also used to prevent recurrences of paroxysmal supraventricular tachycardia. For details of its mode of action, dosage and side effects see pages 45–50.

ii   *Beta blocking drugs* are class II anti-arrhythmics that are used sometimes to convert or prevent recurrences of paroxysmal supraventricular tachycardia or atrial flutter, especially when provoked by exercise, emotion or thyrotoxicosis. For details of the names of some of these drugs, their mode of action, dosage and side effects see page 100.

iii   *Verapamil* is a class IV anti-arrhythmic (calcium antagonist). *Administered intravenously it is the drug most commonly used for the acute conversion of paroxysmal supraventricular tachycardia and atrial flutter to sinus rhythm.* Sometimes it will convert atrial fibrillation of recent onset to sinus rhythm. The intravenous dose of verapamil is 5 mg, repeated once or twice as necessary. Except in high doses, orally verapamil is not a very effective anti-arrhythmic. For details of its mode of action and side effects see page 101.

iv   *Quinidine, disopyramide and flecainide* are drugs of choice for the *prevention* of *recurrent or intermittent* supraventricular tachyarrhythmias such as recurrent atrial fibrillation. As discussed on page 73 they are also used in the treatment of ventricular tachyarrhythmias. As Class I compounds they act by slowing the fast entry of Na^+ ions into the heart muscle cells, thereby slowing the rate of maximum depolarisation. In addition quinidine and disopyramide lengthen the action potential; flecainide has no effect in this respect.

The main side effects of quinidine are that it may induce heart block, and very occasionally in hypersensitive persons may cause cardiac standstill. Disopyramide has mild anti-cholinergic effects and may cause urinary retention. The main side effects of flecainide are dizziness and visual disturbances. Dosage of the drugs is as follows: quinidine 500 mg twice daily, disopyramide 100–200 mg thrice daily, and flecainide 100 mg twice daily.

v   *Amiodarone* is a class III anti-arrhythmic *and is used to treat recurrent arrhythmias not controlled by other drugs*. Its mode of action is to prolong the action potential of heart muscle. Orally it takes about a week to become active. During the first week the oral dose is 200 mg three times a day, gradually reducing thereafter to the minimum dose required to maintain sinus rhythm, usually between 100 mg on alternate days to 200 mg daily. Its main side effects are photosensitivity, interference with thyroid function blood tests, a non-harmful deposition of the drug in the cornea, and diffuse pulmonary alveolitis and hepatitis.

Ventricular tachyarrhythmias
Questions

16i   List the commoner causes of the ventricular arrhythmias.
  ii   Regular rhythms arising in the ventricle are divided into two types according to their speed. Why? What are they? What do they look like on an ECG? How are they treated? As part of your answer, define the term 'ventricular tachycardia'.
  iii   How is ventricular tachycardia distinguished from paroxysmal supraventricular tachycardia with left bundle branch block?

17i   Give a pictorial description of what is happening in the heart, and the ECG changes associated with ventricular fibrillation.
  ii   At what stage after myocardial infarction is ventricular fibrillation most likely to occur?
  iii   Describe the two generally accepted types of ventricular fibrillation.
  iv   How is ventricular fibrillation treated?

Answers

16   **Causes of the ventricular tachyarrhythmias, and the two types of regular ventricular rhythms**

i   The ventricular tachyarrhythmias consist of idioventricular rhythm, ventricular tachycardia and ventricular fibrillation and may be caused by:
  ● Myocardial infarction.
  ● Severe ischaemic heart disease.
  ● Digoxin toxicity, especially in the presence of hypokalaemia.
  ● Cardiomyopathy.
  ● Mitral valve prolapse.
  ● Acquired or congenital prolongation of the QT interval. In

this situation ventricular tachycardia is known as torsades de pointes.

In hospital the ventricular tachyarrhythmias occur most commonly after acute myocardial infarction. In the community they are the commonest cause of sudden death, often occurring in the presence of severe ischaemic heart disease *without* infarction.

ii   Two types of regular ventricular rhythm may occur. Both consist of consecutive ventricular ectopic beats that are recognised on the ECG by the abnormally large wide 'ugly' complexes they produce, duration > 0.12 seconds, and the fact that they are almost always absolutely regular. The two arrhythmias are:
*   *Idioventricular rhythm* with a rate of 60-120 beats per minute. This is usually benign, and as it generally reverts spontaneously to sinus rhythm does not require specific treatment.

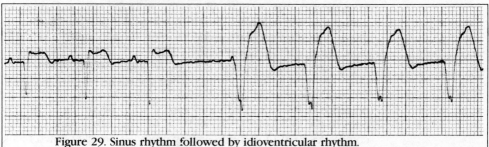

Figure 29. Sinus rhythm followed by idioventricular rhythm.

*   *Ventricular tachycardia.* This is defined simply as three or more consecutive ventricular ectopic beats of the same configuration at a rate greater than about 120 beats per minute. It is most probably due to circular conduction or re-entry similar in principle to that described on page 63.

Ventricular tachycardia may precipitate cardiac failure and is frequently a harbinger of ventricular fibrillation, particularly in the hours and days after acute myocardial infarction. For these reasons it requires immediate treatment. If the patient is tolerating it well it is usual to treat it with intravenous lignocaine 50-100 mg, repeated once if necessary, although other drugs such as disopyramide, mexiletine, flecainide, quinidine and amiodarone may be used. Often lignocaine or one of the other drugs will convert it to sinus rhythm. If it persists, particularly after myocardial infarction, the patient should be sedated with diazepam and cardioverted, using 100-200 joules.

iii   *Differentiation between ventricular tachycardia and supraventricular tachycardia with left bundle branch block.* Left bundle branch block also causes wide complexes, and distinguishing between paroxysmal supraventricular tachycardia with left bundle branch block and ventricular tachycardia may be very difficult. Differentiation is important because intravenous verapamil is dangerous in ventricular tachycardia, often causing

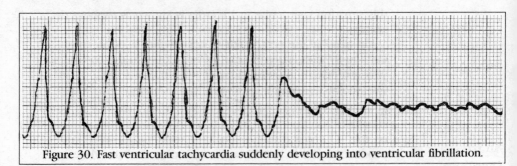

Figure 30. Fast ventricular tachycardia suddenly developing into ventricular fibrillation.

cardiac arrest or hypotension.

Whether the patient appears well or ill cannot be used to differentiate between paroxysmal supraventricular tachycardia and ventricular tachycardia. However, two signs are useful and follow from the fact that in ventricular tachycardia the atria and ventricles contract at different rates. Firstly in ventricular tachycardia the intensity of the first heart sound varies as the atrioventricular valves close intermittently against atrial contraction. Secondly cannon waves may be seen intermittently in the jugular venous pulse as at times the right atrium contracts when the tricuspid valve is closed. Electrocardiographically, ventricular tachycardia is suggested by the presence of P waves (when they can be seen) occurring at different rates to the QRS complexes, and also by particularly wide QRS complexes, > 0.14 seconds, and by gross left bundle branch block.

17   Ventricular fibrillation, the time at which it is most likely to occur after myocardial infarction, its types and treatment

i   Ventricular fibrillation (VF) is probably due to multiple circular currents within the ventricle. With this arrhythmia there is no co-ordinated contraction of the muscle fibres of the ventricles which are therefore shimmering bags of individually contracting muscle fibres. As a consequence VF is associated with lack of any co-ordinated pumping action of the heart, and unless corrected very quickly leads to death. *On the ECG it shows as an unco-ordinated irregular wavy line without any proper complexes.*

ii   VF occurs in about 10% of patients hospitalised with myocardial infarction. Its incidence is greatest in the hours immediately after the infarct, hence the need to hospitalise those patients who are seen early in the course of the illness.

iii   Traditionally VF is divided into two types:
●   *Primary VF.* This is ventricular fibrillation occurring in a patient in whom there is *no preceding heart failure or shock.* Treated properly this type of VF has a relatively good prognosis, and many patients who experience it live to leave hospital.
●   *Secondary VF.* This is ventricular fibrillation occurring in a patient who is *ill with heart failure or shock.* In such cases the prognosis is usually poor.

iv   Treatment of VF:
●   DC defibrillation using 200–400 joules.
●   Since the arrhythmia tends to recur in 10–15% of cases, after defibrillation it is usual to give an anti-arrhythmic drug prophylactically. The standard drug used in this situation is intravenous lignocaine, followed by an oral drug such as disopyramide, mexiletine, flecainide, quinidine or amiodarone for up to 3 months.

An irregular pulse and a fast regular pulse
Questions

18i   List the main causes of an *irregular* pulse.
ii   Assuming you do not have an electrocardiograph, what manoeuvres may be tried to differentiate between them clinically at the bedside?
19   List the causes of a *regular* pulse of 170 beats per minute in a person at rest.

Appendix—pages 76–77

1   A simple plan for sorting out most tachyarrhythmias on an ECG.
2   A simple plan for treating most tachyarrhythmias.

Answers

18   An irregular pulse

i   Main causes are:
●   Atrial or ventricular ectopic beats.
●   Atrial fibrillation.
●   Heart block varying from beat to beat, for instance atrial flutter with variable block, or Wenckebach phenomenon.

ii   Clinical differentiation: if the pulse is basically regular with intermittent irregularities the rhythm is likely to be sinus rhythm with extrasystoles that may be of atrial, junctional or ventricular origin. If the pulse is grossly irregular the rhythm is likely to be atrial fibrillation.
   In cases in which there is difficulty in differentiating between these two alternatives the patient may be gently exercised by, for instance, attempting to touch their toes a few times. In a healthy person in sinus rhythm the speeding of the heart produced by the exercise leaves insufficient time between beats for ectopic beats to be generated. In health the pulse therefore becomes regular as it speeds. By contrast, with atrial fibrillation the tachycardia produced by exercise becomes more irregular as the heart speeds.
   However, when applying this test it is important to appreciate its limitations and to remember that despite underlying sinus rhythm, in the presence of a diseased myocardium, for example due to cardiomyopathy, exercise may increase ectopic activity resulting in a more irregular pulse.

If atrial flutter is suspected the pulse rate may be slowed temporarily by manoeuvres that increase vagal tone such as pressure over the carotid sinus, the Valsalva manoeuvre or pressure over the eyeballs.

19   The causes of a regular pulse of 170 beats per minute in a person at rest

- Paroxysmal supraventricular tachycardia (PSVT) which as discussed on page 63 may be atrial, nodal or related to an accessory bundle.
- Atrial flutter with 2 : 1 block, that is atrial flutter in which alternate beats are conducted to the ventricles.
- Junctional tachycardia.
- Ventricular tachycardia.

Appendix

1   A simple plan for sorting out most tachyarrhythmias on an ECG

Remember there are only six tachyarrhythmias—paroxysmal supraventricular tachycardia, atrial flutter, atrial fibrillation, junctional tachycardia, ventricular tachycardia and ventricular fibrillation.

Look at the tracing and ask the following questions:

- Is it regular or is it irregular?
- Do the ventricular QRS complexes look normal, in which case it is supraventricular, or are they unusually large, wide and 'ugly', duration > 0.12 seconds, in which case it is either ventricular or a supraventricular arrhythmia with left bundle branch block.

Apply the answers to the following plan:

Normal looking QRS complexes = supraventricular arrhythmia

Regular:

- Paroxysmal supraventricular tachycardia, or
- Atrial flutter with regular block, or
- Junctional tachycardia

Differentiation of these may be helped by looking for P waves, and if present, by timing their relationship to the QRS complexes.

Irregular:

- Atrial fibrillation, or
- Atrial flutter with variable block

Abnormally large wide 'ugly' QRS complexes = ventricular arrhythmia or paroxysmal supraventricular tachycardia with left bundle branch block

Regular:

● Ventricular tachycardia, or
● Paroxysmal supraventricular tachycardia with left bundle branch block

Irregular:

● Ventricular fibrillation, or
● Atrial fibrillation with left bundle branch block or the Wolff-Parkinson-White syndrome.

2   A simple plan for treating most tachyarrhythmias

	Acute	*Long-term*
Supraventricular		
● Paroxysmal supra-ventricular tachycardia* ● Atrial flutter	Verapamil i.v. (Ill patient— ? DC shock)	Flecainide Disopyramide Quinidine Beta blocker** Amiodarone***
● Atrial fibrillation	Digitalis (Recent onset—? DC shock)	Digitalis
Ventricular		
● Ventricular tachycardia	Lignocaine i.v. DC shock (± overdrive pacing for recurrent cases)	Flecainide Disopyramide Quinidine Amiodarone**
● Ventricular fibrillation	Blow on chest Defibrillation	

* First try Valsalva manoeuvre.
** For cases associated with emotion, exercise or thyrotoxicosis.
*** For cases resistant to the other drugs.

Further Reading

Braunwald E (ed) (1984). *Heart Disease*, 2nd edition. WB Saunders, Philadelphia. Chapters 19, mechanisms and diagnosis of arrhythmias; 20, management of arrhythmias.
Hampton JR (1986) *The ECG Made Easy*, 3rd edition. Churchill Livingstone, Edinburgh.

Four Cases of Chest Pain

Case C   # A Case of Chest Pain— No. 1: Mrs B-D, aged 63 years

An anxious widowed lady who tends to worry about her unhappily married only son, and lives alone in a privately rented first floor apartment with no lift.

History of present condition

Complaining for 4 years of pains across the chest, worse in the last 3 months, now occurring more than once per day.

Past medical history

Inferior myocardial infarct 9 months previously.
Arthritis in the back and knees for 5 years.
Hysterectomy for fibroids 13 years previously.
Laparotomy 15 years previously.
Hypertension 32 years.

Relevant direct questions

Shortness of breath: with chest pain only.
Swelling of ankles: nil.
Palpitations: nil.
Smoking: smoked 20 cigarettes per day until 5 years previously.
Drugs: Slow release oxprenolol 160 mg daily for 4 years.
Nitroglycerin 0.5 mg sublingually as required.
Aspirin as required for arthritic pains.

Examination

Small overweight pale middle-aged lady in whom examination of all systems was normal.
BP 160/90 lying, 140/70 standing.

Comment on the history

Mrs B-D was not very forthcoming and her initial history was not very helpful in suggesting the cause of her pain. This posed a problem as in general the diagnosis is suggested by the history more commonly than by any other diagnostic manoeuvre.

On page 4 the importance was stressed of using one's imagination when taking the history, of imagining oneself to be the patient, sharing their experience, establishing the time of day, where the patient was and what they were doing when their complaint began. As we shall see, by applying these principles Mrs B-D was found to have no less than three different chest pains.

Mrs B-D

Questions

1   Read the following history of each of Mrs B-D's chest pains. What do you think was the cause of each pain?

Substernal chest pain no. 1

This pain had been present for 4 years. It occurred on climbing stairs, walking on the flat in the cold and also when she was worried about her son. It radiated to the left arm. It was eased within 5 minutes by rest, and within 1–2 minutes by nitroglycerin. Currently, it was occurring with increasing frequency, more than once a day, after walking about 250 yards on the flat.

Substernal chest pain no. 2

Although this pain radiated to the arm, it was different from substernal pain no. 1, as it occurred within a few minutes of eating and on lying flat, and was relieved by Gaviscon, a mixture of alginic acid and antacids, and also like substernal pain no. 1, by sublingual nitroglycerin. It had been present for 4 years.

Substernal chest pain no. 3

This was a sharp non-radiating pain that had started following a fall 18 months before. It was worse with coughing, bending, reaching up and carrying weights in the left hand. It was eased by keeping still. Generally, it lasted only a few minutes, but on occasion might last for many hours or days.

2   Mrs B-D was described as 'overweight'. Define the terms 'overweight' and 'obesity'.

3   Why do you think Mrs B-D's blood pressure dropped a little when she changed from the lying to the standing position?

Answers

1   Mrs B-D's chest pains

No. 1 was typical of angina due to ischaemic heart disease.
No. 2 was typical of oesophageal pain and in fact was due to a
hiatus hernia demonstrated by barium meal. Note that like angina,
oesophageal pain may radiate to the arm, and that also like angina,
spasm of oesophageal smooth muscle may be relieved by
nitroglycerin.
No. 3 was musculoskeletal, and was demonstrated by pressing
on the sternum. It is important to explain to the patient that
although this type of pain may last for months or even years it is
usually of no great clinical or prognostic significance.

2   Definitions of overweight and obesity

Overweight is defined as weighing 110–119% of one's acceptable
or standard weight.
Obesity is defined as weighing 120% or more of one's
acceptable or standard weight.
    Acceptable or standard weight is based on two large studies in
the United States in which weight and mortality were studied over
many years in several million insurance policy holders.

3   Change of blood pressure with posture

Normally, on standing the pulse pressure temporarily narrows as
the systolic pressure falls and the diastolic pressure rises. In Mrs B-
D's case the fall in the blood pressure when she stood was
probably due to the oxprenolol (a beta blocker) she was taking for
hypertension. On occasion most of the drugs used in the treatment
of hypertension cause postural hypotension. Autonomic
neuropathy, due for instance to diabetes mellitus, may also cause
postural hypotension, as may dehydration, or simply being ill. It is
therefore good clinical practice to take the blood pressure of every
patient in the lying and standing positions. In patients receiving
treatment for hypertension it is mandatory to do so.

Chapter 4
Differential Diagnosis of Chest Pain

Questions

1   List the direct questions that should be asked about the characteristics of any pain in order to elucidate its cause; for example where is it, how long has it been present?
2   List the additional direct questions that should be asked to differentiate chest pain due to the gastrointestinal tract, the chest wall or the skeletal system, the heart, the pleura; for example does it occur with coughing, is it eased by antacid?
3   What techniques or manoeuvres can you apply when examining a patient to test whether or not their chest pain is of musculoskeletal origin?
4   Chest pain may arise from many organs within the chest, and also from distant organs such as the brain or psyche. For each organ list all the common causes of chest pain, giving a brief description of each. Include short descriptions of Bornholm disease (epidemic myalgia), and Tietze's syndrome.

Answers

1   The direct questions that should be asked about any pain

- Where is it?
- How long has it been present?
- Did it start in relationship to any particular event such as a fall or other trauma, reaching up, a previous heart attack?
- What does it feel like, i.e. what is its character?
- Does it radiate, and if so, where?
- How long does it last?
- What brings it on or makes it worse?
- What relieves it?
- How frequently does it occur?

Although these questions seem very simple and basic, it is surprising how often in practice the correct diagnosis is missed because they were not asked.

2   The additional questions that should be asked about a case of chest pain

Is it brought on by:

Eating
Bending forwards
Swallowing
Lying flat
} Suggesting pain from the oesophagus or gastrointestinal tract

Bending
Twisting
Reaching up
Using the arms
Taking a deep breath
Coughing
Lying on one side
Pressure over the affected area
} Suggesting pain of musculoskeletal origin

Walking, hurrying
Climbing hills
Going out in the cold
Excitement, anxiety or anger
} Suggesting angina or cardiac pain

Taking a deep breath
Coughing
Twisting
Pressure over the affected area
} Suggesting pleuritic pain

Is it relieved by:

● *Rest*—suggestive of angina although it should be remembered that musculoskeletal pain may also be eased by rest.
● *Keeping the chest as still as possible*—suggestive of both pleurisy and musculoskeletal pain.
● *Nitroglycerin*—suggestive of angina although it should be remembered that nitroglycerin also relaxes oesophageal smooth muscle thereby sometimes relieving pain due to oesophageal spasm.
● *Antacids*—suggestive of pain from the upper gastrointestinal tract.

3   Techniques or manoeuvres that may be employed when examining a patient to test whether or not the pain is of musculoskeletal origin

Test whether the pain is reproduced by:
● Coughing.
● Bending, stretching, twisting.
● Pressing over the affected area.
● Opposing abduction, adduction, extension and flexion of the arms and shoulders.

Comment

The importance of performing these manoeuvres is amply demonstrated by the following case.

Mrs C-H, a 62 year old housewife, who smoked 15 cigarettes a day, was admitted to a coronary care unit with a suspected myocardial infarct following exacerbation of chest pain that had been present for 9 months and had been treated as angina with nitroglycerin, nifedipine and propranolol. A careful history revealed that although the pain occurred with exertion it was sited to the left of the sternum and radiated up over the pectoral muscles and down under the left breast. An electrocardiograph was normal throughout an exercise test. A chest x-ray was also normal. The pain was reproduced by pressing on the sternum and opposing abduction of the arms. The patient was greatly relieved when the musculoskeletal nature of the pain was explained to her. She was advised to stop smoking, her anti-anginal therapy was stopped and she resumed a normal life. Presumably, the pain occurred with walking because of swinging of the arms.

4   The commoner causes of chest pain

From the heart (all typically felt in the centre of the chest)

● *Angina pectoris.* Typically angina pectoris is a tight, crushing or constricting pain that is precipitated by exertion, and relieved by rest. In about half the cases it radiates to one or both arms, the throat or jaw.
● *Myocardial infarction.* The pain of myocardial infarction is generally a severe anginal-like pain that occurs at rest or persists after exertion despite rest.
● *Pericarditis.* Typically the pain of pericarditis is a central pleuritic-like chest pain that is worse lying flat, and eased by sitting up, or adopting some other particular position.

From the aorta

● *Dissecting aneurysm.* The pain of a dissecting aneurysm is often described as a severe tearing pain that moves up to the neck and then down the front or back of the trunk as the dissection proceeds.

From the lungs

● *Pleurisy.* Pain from the pleura is usually described as a sharp unilateral pain that varies with coughing and breathing. The commonest causes of pleural pain are infection that may be within the pleura or secondary to pneumonia, pulmonary embolus with infarction, or carcinoma of the bronchus involving the pleura.
● *Spontaneous pneumothorax.* Typically this pain is described as a tearing unilateral pain that is sometimes accompanied by breathlessness.
● *Pancoast tumour.* This pain is due to a carcinoma at the apex of the lung invading the brachial plexus and adjacent ribs, and is usually described as an unremitting severe pain over the top of one shoulder and down the arm.

- *Tracheobronchitis.* This pain is usually described as a raw central chest pain that is often worse with coughing and breathing, and is typically due to viral infections or inhalation of a noxious vapour.

From the oesophagus

Typically pain from the oesophagus is described as a tight indigestion-like pain in the centre of the chest. The main causes of oesophageal pain are:

- *Oesophageal spasm* due to regurgitation of food or acid.
- *Oesophagitis* due to inflammation of the lower oesophagus caused by the regurgitation of food and acid.
- *Inco-ordinate tertiary muscle contractions.* Typically this occurs in the middle-aged and elderly and may be related to food or occur spontaneously.
- *Dysphagia* (difficulty with swallowing) due to:
a   Stricture of the oesophagus.
b   Hiatus hernia.
c   Trapped foreign body such as a bone.
- *Carcinoma of the oesophagus*, or less commonly invasion of the oesophagus by a carcinoma of the bronchus.
- *Oesophageal rupture.* Usually this occurs after vomiting, and typically is described as a deep severe pain.

From the musculoskeletal system

Pain of this type is usually localised and of a sharp pleuritic nature. The causes of musculoskeletal chest pain are:

- *Torn muscle fibres.*
- *Cracked or fractured ribs*—due to trauma, or spontaneous in association with osteoporosis or metastatic carcinoma.
- *Metastases* growing within a rib.
- *Osteoarthritis* of the costosternal joints, that is, as shown in Figure 31, osteoarthritis of the synovial joints between the sternum and the rib cartilages.
- *Osteochondritis or Tietze's syndrome*, which is a condition characterised by painful swelling of one or more of the upper costochondrial joints that as shown in Figure 31 are the non-synovial joints between the ribs and rib cartilages.
- *Epidemic myalgia or Bornholm disease*, which is a condition characterised by fever and severe unilateral chest pain associated with focal necrosis of the muscles of the chest wall as a result of infection with a Coxsackie B virus.
- *Frozen shoulder.* Also known as adhesive capsulitis, this condition is typified by pain in the area of the shoulder on moving or lying on the arm, and is due to inflammation with or without fibrotic thickening of the glenohumeral joint.
- *Referred pain* from the cervical or thoracic spine, or from a costovertebral angle.

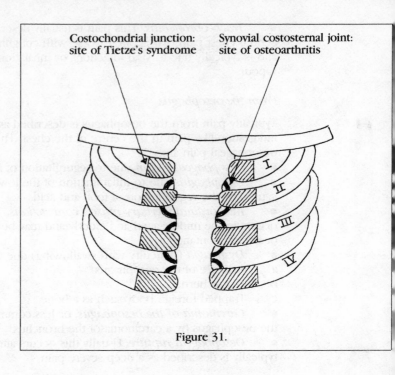

Costochondral junction:
site of Tietze's syndrome

Synovial costosternal joint:
site of osteoarthritis

Figure 31.

From the skin

The conditions associated with pain from the skin are unilateral, namely:

● *Herpes zoster (shingles)*. Because the pain of shingles may precede the rash by a day or so, unless it is considered in the differential diagnosis of unilateral chest pain, chest pain due to shingles may be misdiagnosed.

● *Post-herpetic neuralgia*. This is a condition characterised by chronic pain localised to a dermatome in which the sensory nerves have been damaged by a previous attack of shingles.

From the abdomen

Disease of several viscera in the upper abdomen may cause pain in the chest. The commonest are:

● *Peptic ulcer*
● *Biliary colic*
● *Diaphragmatic pain*. Often pain from the diaphragm is felt in the shoulder as well as in the abdomen. The explanation of this is that both areas are innervated by nerves from the same dermatome (C4), and that pain in the diaphragm is perceived in the shoulder in much the same way, as explained on page 90, that angina is felt in the arm.

From the psyche

- *Da Costa's syndrome.* This is described on page 93.
- *Hyperventilation.* Overbreathing may produce typical anginal-like pain in a percentage of persons both with and without ischaemic heart disease, and is an important but usually overlooked cause of anginal pain unrelated to exercise. Dizziness and tingling of the fingers and feet are useful pointers to a diagnosis of hyperventilation.

Chapter 5
Angina Pectoris

Pathology; the coronary circulation; electrocardiograph leads

Questions

1i   Name the four types of cells involved in the pathogenesis of
the atherosclerotic lesion, and write a brief note about the role of
each in the development of such a lesion.
ii   Give a brief description of a fatty streak and a fibrous plaque.
iii   At which sites in the arterial tree is atherosclerosis most
likely to have important clinical consequences?
2   Why is angina felt in the centre and not on the left side of
the chest? What is the accepted explanation of why cardiac pain is
felt in the arms?
3i   Draw a simple diagram of the coronary circulation, naming
the main coronary arteries. Superimpose on the diagram which
surface of the heart each of the two main coronary arteries
supplies. Also superimpose on the diagram the positions of the
various ECG leads.
ii   In addition to the diagram, write a brief note stating the
areas of the heart supplied by (a) the left coronary artery, and (b)
the right coronary artery.
iii   Which ECG leads reflect events in: (a) the anteroseptal area
of the heart, (b) the anterior surface of the heart, (c) the
anterolateral surface of the heart, (d) the inferior surface of the
heart.

Answers

**1i   The four types of cells involved in the pathogenesis of
the atherosclerotic lesion**

Although the pathogenesis of the atherosclerotic lesion is not fully
understood, it is known that four types of cells are involved.
●   *Arterial endothelial cells*. The atherosclerotic process is
thought to be initiated as a result of injury to these cells by low
density and other lipoproteins that bind to the cell membrane and
pass into the subendothelial space. Alternative possibilities are that
endothelial cells are damaged by mechanical trauma, toxins or
viruses.
●   *Leucocytes, mainly monocytes*. It has long been known that
blood monocytes give rise to tissue macrophages or histiocytes. In
the atherosclerotic process monocytes appear to be attracted by
chemotactic substances elaborated by injured endothelial cells to

which they adhere before migrating subendothelially between the endothelial cells, binding lipoprotein and becoming lipid laden macrophages (foam cells).

● *Smooth muscle cells*. Under the influence of chemotactic substances elaborated by the other cells smooth muscle cells proliferate and migrate from the media to the intima of the arterial wall.

● *Platelets*. These are involved in the atherosclerotic process in at least two ways. Firstly, by producing substances such as platelet derived growth factor (PDGF), a small protein, about 30 000 daltons that affects the migration of other cells within the vessel wall, platelets appear to be directly involved in the growth of the atherosclerotic lesion. Secondly, platelets become attached to lesions over which the endothelium has broken exposing small areas of subendothelium.

1ii   Fatty streaks and fibrous plaques

Fatty streaks are the earliest atherosclerotic lesion, and occur in young children. They are situated in the subendothelial area, and consist predominantly of lipd laden macrophages derived mainly from blood monocytes, together with some smooth muscle cells that have migrated from the media.

Fibrous plaques are more advanced lesions and consist of smooth muscle cells that have migrated to the intima, and lipid laden macrophages surrounded by a matrix of connective tissue and variable amounts of intra- and extracellular lipids. Over the top of the lesion is a dense cap of smooth muscle cells and fibrous

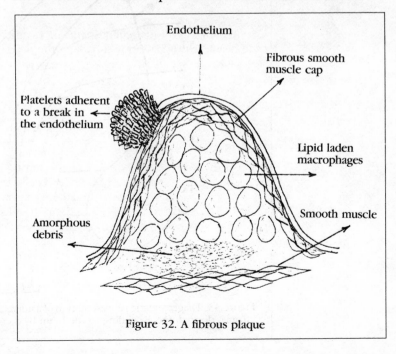

Figure 32. A fibrous plaque

tissue. Beneath the lesion there may be an area of necrosis, cholesterol crystals and calcification. If the layer of endothelial cells covering the lesion has broken there may be adhesion of platelets and thrombus formation.

Fibrous plaques protrude into the lumen of an artery. Pieces may rupture from a plaque, or break off as a result of blood burrowing into the vessel wall beneath the plaque. Platelet aggregation and frank intra-arterial thrombosis may occur on the roughened and broken surface of a plaque. These events lead to narrowing of the vessel's lumen and ischaemia which may stimulate small nerve fibres with production of the sensation we know as pain.

1iii   The arterial sites at which atherosclerosis is most likely to have important clinical consequences

●   The coronary arteries
●   The cerebral arteries
●   The ilio/femoral/popliteal arteries
●   The bifurcation of the common carotid arteries
●   The abdominal aorta

2   The distribution of anginal pain

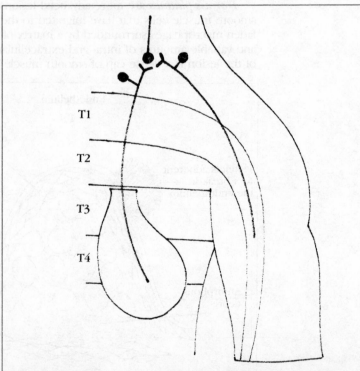

Figure 33. Diagrammatic representation of a nerve from the heart and from a dermatome ascending to the brain by a common pathway

Angina is felt in the centre of the chest because the heart is a midline organ with mediastinal attachments.

Angina is felt in the arms and across the chest and sometimes in the neck because embryologically the heart is derived from the same dermatomes as the inner sides of the arms and the upper chest, namely dermatomes C7-T4. The sensory nerves from the heart run back centrally along the sympathetic nerves that run out to the heart. One explanation of the fact that heart pain is felt across the chest and in the arms is that within the central nervous system sensory nerves from both the heart and the arms ascend in the same pathways to the brain.

3   The coronary circulation and ECG leads

i

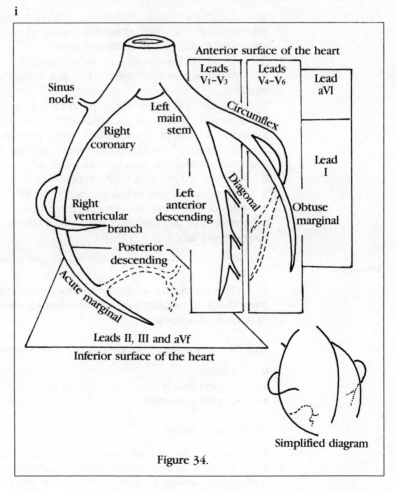

Figure 34.

ii(a)   The *left coronary artery* supplies the anterior, lateral and part of the posterior walls of the left ventricle, and the antero-superior two-thirds of the interventricular septum.

ii(b)   The *right coronary artery* runs in the atrioventricular groove to supply the inferior border of the left ventricle, part of the posterior wall of the left ventricle, the right ventricle, the sinus node, and the postero-inferior third of the interventricular septum.

iii   ECG leads and sites of ischaemia:

Site	ECG lead
• Anteroseptal	V_1–V_3
• Anterior	V_1–V_6
• Anterolateral	V_4–V_6, I and aVl
• Inferior	II, III, aVf

Contributing factors; clinical syndromes

Questions

4   List the treatable underlying conditions, such as hypertension, that may contribute to angina and which should always be looked for in a case of angina.

5   Describe Prinzmetal's or variant angina.

6   What is unstable angina? Why is it dangerous? How is it treated?

7   Despite exclusion of the potentially treatable underlying conditions such as anaemia, hypertension and valvular disease listed in the answer to question 4, some patients with troublesome anginal-like pain have normal coronary arteries. List the main causes of anginal-like pain in such patients.

8   Describe Da Costa's syndrome.

9   In patients with ischaemic heart disease what percentage of episodes of ischaemia are associated with pain and what percentage are painless? At what time of day do peak numbers of episodes occur?

Answers

4   The treatable underlying conditions that may contribute to angina and which should always be looked for in a case of angina

Risk factors for the development of atherosclerosis

• Smoking
• Hypertension
• Hyperlipidaemia

Cardiac conditions

• Aortic valve disease, particularly aortic stenosis
• Paroxysmal arrhythmias, either supraventricular or ventricular, causing a rapid pulse and low blood pressure

Other conditions

• Diabetes mellitus
• Anaemia

- Hypothyroidism, and less commonly thyrotoxicosis
- Obesity

5 Prinzmetal's or variant angina

The original description of this was of angina at rest with transient ST elevation due to spasm in an atherosclerotic coronary artery. It is now appreciated that angina at rest may occur with spasm of a normal as well as an atherosclerotic coronary artery and that it may be associated with transient ST depression as well as transient ST elevation.

6 Unstable angina

This is worsening angina or angina occurring at rest. Synonyms for unstable angina are crescendo angina and pre-infarction syndrome. The danger of unstable angina is that it is likely to lead to myocardial infarction. Vigorous treatment is therefore indicated, including bed rest, adequate analgesia with opiates if necessary, administration of oral aspirin and the drugs mentioned in the answers to questions 17-20, and possibly anticoagulation with heparin. Although unproven by formal trial, it is generally agreed that patients with unstable angina that does not settle in a few hours with full medical treatment should proceed to urgent coronary arteriography, and if indicated, coronary artery bypass surgery or angioplasty.

7 Anginal-like pain in patients with normal coronary arteries

Despite exclusion of the potentially treatable underlying conditions listed in the answer to question 4, some patients who undergo coronary arteriograms for apparently typical angina of effort are shown to have normal coronary arteries. In these cases the cause of the pain is thought to be:
- Temporary spasm of a coronary artery.
- Hyperventilation during exercise or at other times causing spasm of a coronary artery.
- Gastric reflux occurring during exercise and causing a pain similar to angina of effort.
- Pain from the skeleton or some other organ.

A clue to the cause of this type of angina is that often it is brought on by variable rather than fairly consistent levels of exertion. Treatment is that of the underlying condition. Nifedipine may help some patients with coronary artery spasm.

8 Da Costa's syndrome

This is chest pain of psychological origin in a patient with an anxious personality. Classically patients with Da Costa's syndrome are said to adopt a stooping or even apologetic posture. Typically they complain of exhaustion and breathlessness at rest or on minimal exertion, and of palpitations, and dizziness that is probably due to hyperventilation. The chest pain is usually over the left breast, and is of a sharp or pricking character, lasting from a few seconds to several hours.

9 Percentages of painful and painless episodes of ischaemia

Continuous recording of the ECG in patients with ischaemic heart disease has shown that about 25% of episodes of ischaemic ST depression are associated with anginal-like pain and that about 75% of episodes are painless or silent. Most episodes occur during the day (as opposed to the night) with peak numbers about the time of waking in the morning, and also in the early evening. The morning peak coincides with the diurnal morning peak of catecholamine release, plasma cortisol, heart rate, blood pressure, onset of myocardial infarction and sudden cardiac death.

Investigation (i)
Questions

10 List the specific investigations that should be ordered in a case of angina. What are the abnormalities they may show?
11 Draw the different patterns of ECG changes that may be seen with cardiac ischaemia (as opposed to myocardial infarction).
12 What is the likelihood of a resting ECG being normal in a patient with a history of angina but no actual pain at the time of the recording?

Answers

10 The specific investigations of a case of angina

These have two main purposes:
● To establish the correct diagnosis, the severity of the condition and the need for treatment.
● To identify any contributing factors such as hyperlipidaemia, anaemia or hypothyroidism.

The following tests are normally performed:
● *Haemoglobin (Hb)*, to assess whether the patient is anaemic or polycythaemic.
● *Fasting lipids*. These may be measured for two reasons:
a To determine if the patient has a hyperlipidaemia that might respond to treatment with slowing of the progression of their atheromatous disease. Generally this is less rewarding in persons aged over 65 years, and because of this, the test is less often performed in these patients.
b To determine if the patient has a familial hyperlipidaemia for which younger members of their family should be screened and possibly treated prophylactically.
● *Thyroid function tests*, usually only if clinically indicated.
● *Resting ECG*, to assess any changes that might indicate ischaemia, or previous myocardial infarction.

- *Exercise ECG with or without thallium scintigraphy*, if indicated (discussed in the answers to questions 13-16).
- *Coronary arteriography*, if indicated (see page 102).

11   ECG changes in ischaemia

Cardiac ischaemia produces changes in the ST segment or T wave of the ECG. ST depression, or inversion or flattening of the T wave, is due to endocardial ischaemia, and ST elevation to epicardial or transmural ischaemia.

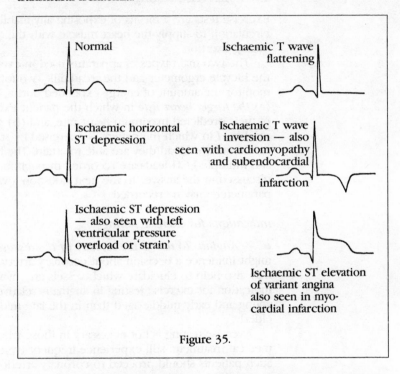

Normal

Ischaemic T wave flattening

Ischaemic horizontal ST depression

Ischaemic T wave inversion — also seen with cardiomyopathy and subendocardial infarction

Ischaemic ST depression — also seen with left ventricular pressure overload or 'strain'

Ischaemic ST elevation of variant angina also seen in myocardial infarction

Figure 35.

NOTE: ST depression may also be caused by digitalis, and T wave inversion or flattening may also be caused by hypokalaemia.

12   The resting ECG in a patient with a history of angina, but no actual pain at the time of recording

The resting ECG is likely to be normal in about 75% of patients with a history of angina. However, in most of these it becomes abnormal if they are sufficiently exercised or stressed.

Investigation (ii): exercise testing; thallium scintigraphy
Questions

13   In a sentence or two describe the two types of apparatus used in exercise testing, and the two ways that the effort expended during the test is monitored. What are the indications for exercise testing?

14 List and write short notes on the various parameters or end points that may be monitored to assess an exercise test.
15 Some of these parameters are more sensitive and specific than others. Define the terms 'sensitivity' and 'specificity'.
16 What is thallium scintigraphy of the heart? Describe the four main patterns of results it may yield.

Answers

13 Exercise testing

Exercise tests are a means of exposing any inability of the coronary circulation to supply the heart muscle with the oxygen it needs during exertion.

The two main types of apparatus used in exercise testing are the bicycle ergometer and the treadmill. Two formats are used to monitor the amount of energy expended during the test, namely (a) *the target heart rate* in which the patient exercises to 80–90% of their predicted maximum heart rate, and (b) *the maximum workload* in which the patient is exercised by stages to the maximum workload they are able to attain. The blood pressure and multiple ECG leads are recorded throughout the test. As discussed in the answer to the next question a variety of parameters may be recorded.

Indications for exercise testing

● *Angina. To assess the severity of the disease*, particularly if it might influence a decision about coronary artery bypass surgery. It may also help to elucidate which vessels are involved. The indication for exercise testing in angina is relatively stronger in the young and early middle-aged than in the late middle-aged and elderly.

Exercise testing is not necessary in those who, despite proper medical treatment, still experience frequent typical angina of effort. Such patients should proceed to coronary arteriography.

● *A diagnostic procedure* where angina is a possible cause of chest pain of unknown aetiology, so called atypical chest pain.

● *After myocardial infarction* to help assess the need for coronary artery bypass as there is evidence that the individuals most likely to die or have a further infarct after a myocardial infarction are those who develop anginal-like pain or ECG changes of ischaemia on exercise. In one study the mortality in the first year after infarction was 27% in those with exercise induced ST changes, and only 2% in those without. Again, the indication for exercise testing in this situation is relatively stronger in the young than in the elderly.

14 The parameters that may be monitored to assess an exercise test

The specificity of these varies, and is affected by the number of risk factors for ischaemic heart disease in the person being tested. Thus the occurrence of chest pain during the test is more likely to be due to ischaemic heart disease in a 60 year old hypertensive male smoker with a high serum cholesterol than a 30 year old normotensive female non-smoker with a normal serum cholesterol. In Western societies where other conditions that might give a positive result, such as cardiomyopathy, are rare, *the development of anginal-like chest pain and significant ECG changes* at lower than normal workloads or at low heart rates are the most specific parameters of coronary artery disease, yielding a positive result in about 80% of cases.

With this in mind the parameters that may be monitored during an exercise test are:

● *Poor exercise tolerance.* Stopping the test because of dyspnoea or exhaustion. Clearly this criterion is non-specific, and may reflect disease of other systems such as the respiratory system, or even unwillingness to continue the test rather than inability to complete it.

● *The development of anginal pain.* As stated above, this is suggestive of cardiac ischaemia, but of course pain is a subjective phenomenon that cannot be measured directly.

● *The development of ischaemic ST depression on the ECG.* The *sensitivity* of the test (ability to detect the disease) may be increased by using fairly minor ST depression as a criterion of ischaemia, for example 1 mm (0.1 mV). The *specificity* of the test (ability to differentiate between diseases) is increased by adopting stricter criteria, for example ST depression 2 mm (0.2 mV.).

● *Increase in the amplitude of the R wave.* Although it may be affected by other factors, in general the height of the R wave reflects left ventricular size. In healthy persons the left ventricle empties more completely during exercise, becomes smaller and as a consequence produces a smaller R wave. In persons with a diseased heart the volume of the left ventricle and the size of the R wave usually increase on exercise.

● *Fall of blood pressure.* In healthy persons the blood pressure rises with exercise. In persons with poor left ventricular function it either fails to rise or falls.

● *The development of ectopic beats or more serious arrhythmias.* In healthy persons sinus tachycardia suppresses any such activity.

Severe disease is indicated by early onset of anginal-like pain, or slow recovery, marked and widespread ST depression, a falling blood pressure, or the development of arrhythmias.

15 'Sensitivity' and 'Specificity'

● *Sensitivity* is the ability of a relevant test to detect a disease. Clearly, the lower or easier the criteria of the test, the more cases will be detected, the greater will be the sensitivity of the test, and the fewer the false negatives (missed cases).

● *Specificity* is the ability of a test to differentiate the disease being investigated from other diseases. The specificity of a test is increased by raising the level of criteria used, resulting in few false positives (cases wrongly diagnosed because of undemanding criteria).

16   Thallium scintigraphy of the heart

The specificity of exercise testing may be increased and further information about the state of the coronary arteries obtained by performing thallium-201 scintigraphy when the end point of the exercise test is reached. Thallium-201 is injected intravenously and is distributed in the tissues in a similar way to potassium. It is rapidly distributed to well perfused myocardium, less well to areas of ischaemia, and usually not at all to areas of acute or past

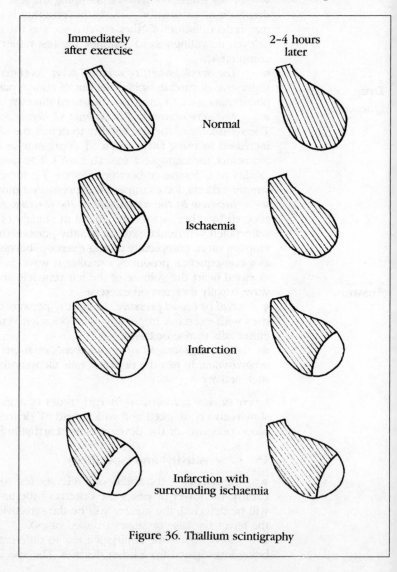

Figure 36. Thallium scintigraphy

infarction. Scans are taken immediately and repeated 2-4 hours later. Four main patterns are recognised:
- *Normal*. Distribution of isotope to all areas of the myocardium.
- *Ischaemia*. A reversible pattern of poor perfusion of ischaemic areas immediately after the test due to the effects of exercise, with distribution of the isotope to ischaemic areas by the time the test is repeated 2-4 hours later.
- *Infarction*. A non-reversible pattern of poor perfusion due to isotope not being distributed to the infarcted area.
- *Infarction with surrounding ischaemia*. An area of non-reversible poor perfusion surrounded by an area with reversible perfusion.

The sensitivity of the test is limited by the need to compare one area with another, and the fact that diffuse or widespread ischaemia may not produce areas of sufficient contrast for interpretation.

Drug treatment
Questions

17 What are the aims, so far as the circulation and function of the heart are concerned, of the drug treatment of angina?
18 How is nitroglycerin thought to work? What are its main side effects?
19 Name three or four beta blocking drugs and give their typical daily doses. How are beta blockers thought to act? What are their main side effects?
20 Name three calcium channel blocking drugs. How are calcium channel blockers thought to act? What are their main side effects?

Answers

17 The aims of drug treatment

These are to relieve the pain and if possible improve the prognosis of the condition by:
- Reducing myocardial oxygen consumption.
- Increasing the blood supply along the coronary arteries if possible.

18 The actions of nitroglycerin and its side effects

Nitroglycerin is taken sublingually by tablet or spray for the relief of acute attacks of angina, and most importantly, *prophylactically before* any activity likely to precipitate an attack.
Its main actions are:
- *Reduction of the work and oxygen consumption of the heart due to:*
a *Venous dilatation* causing pooling of blood in veins such as those of the limbs, and as a result, a reduction of preload.

b   *Arterial dilatation*. With small doses of nitroglycerin this is less prominent than venous dilatation. However, arterial dilation may occur with the amount of nitroglycerin in an 0.5 mg tablet, resulting in hypotension and reduction of afterload.

●   *Direct dilatation of the coronary arteries*. In most cases the atherosclerotic process probably prevents this. In some cases, however, collateral vessels may respond and dilate with benefit.

The main side effects of nitroglycerin are:

●   *Pulsation in the head or headache* due to vasodilatation of the blood vessels supplying the head.

●   *Dizziness or even syncope* due to rapid lowering of the blood pressure.

NOTE: Long-acting nitrates may be taken sublingually, as a tablet laid against the buccal mucosa, orally by absorption from the upper gastrointestinal tract, and by absorption through the skin via an impregnated patch or ointment. However, tolerance and lack of efficacy develops in up to 40% of users, but may be overcome by omitting the medication overnight for about 10-12 hours.

19   The names and daily dosages of several beta blockers, their mode of action and main side effects

There are over a dozen beta blockers on the market. Examples are:

Cardioselective: blocking mainly ß1 adrenoreceptors
●   Atenolol: 50-100 mg once daily.
●   Metoprolol: up to about 400 mg daily in divided doses.

Non-cardioselective: blocking ß1 + ß2 adrenoreceptors
●   Propranolol: up to 320 mg daily in divided doses.
●   Sotalol: 80-200 mg once daily.
●   Oxprenolol: up to 320 mg daily in divided doses.

Mode of action

Beta blocking drugs act by competitively inhibiting the actions of catecholamines on post-synaptic beta receptors. In angina their main action is to reduce myocardial oxygen consumption, particularly on exercise by slowing the heart (negative chronotropic effect) and by reducing the power of contraction of the cardiac muscle (negative inotropic effect) resulting in a reduction of cardiac work and cardiac output.

Main side effects

●   *Bradycardia*. Pulse < 50 beats per minute, or even heart block on occasion.

●   *Precipitation of cardiac failure* due to their negative inotropic effect and the bradycardia. A history of cardiac failure is usually a contraindication to the use of beta blockers.

●   *Asthma* due to blockade of ß2 bronchodilator receptors in the lungs. Beta blockers may precipitate severe asthma in known asthmatics and may also worsen chronic obstructive airways disease. They are therefore contraindicated in these conditions. Even Timóptol eye drops, containing about 0.2 mg timolol per drop, may precipitate a fatal asthmatic attack in known asthmatics.

● *Raynaud's phenomenon* due to reduction of cardiac output and blockade of vasodilator ß2 sympathetic receptors in the walls of arterioles.

● *Feelings of fatigue* possibly due to reduction of cardiac output.

● *Bad dreams*. These are said to occur mainly with those beta blockers that are lipophilic, that is highly fat soluble and thus more soluble in the brain, than with those that are hydrophilic, that is highly water soluble.

● *Impotence*. This is increased by about a third and should be enquired about in all male patients taking beta blockers.

● *Hypotension* due to reduction of cardiac output.

20   The names of three calcium channel blocking drugs, their modes of action and side effects

Action

These drugs act by inhibiting the influx of calcium ions into myocardial muscle and vascular smooth muscle cells. This results in reduced activity of the enzyme ATPase within these cells, causing:

● *Reduced contractility of the heart muscle cells* resulting in reduction of cardiac work and output and oxygen consumption by the heart.

● *Relaxation of arterial smooth muscle* in the periphery resulting in reduction of afterload.

● *Relaxation of the coronary vascular smooth muscle* of those coronary arteries that are not irreversibly stenosed. This makes these drugs particularly useful in the treatment of angina due to coronary artery spasm.

The three most frequently used calcium channel blocking drugs

● *Nifedipine* in divided doses from 15 mg per day up to a maximum of about 60 mg per day. The main side effects of nifedipine are dizziness, flushing and headache due to arterial dilatation and also oedema of the legs probably due to an increase in permeability of small blood vessels.

● *Verapamil* in divided doses from 120 to 360 mg per day. The main side effects of verapamil are constipation, and occasionally conduction problems within the heart that may even cause heart block, especially if the drug is used with a beta blocker—a combination that can be dangerous.

● *Diltiazem* in divided doses, usually about 180 mg per day, although occasionally patients may require up to 480 mg per day.

The main side effects of diltiazem are nausea, bradycardia, first degree heart block, oedema of the legs, swelling of the fingers and occasionally, rashes.

Coronary arteriography and coronary artery bypass surgery

Questions

21   What is coronary arteriography? What are the indications for performing it?

22i   In a few sentences describe what coronary artery bypass is, and the various surgical techniques by which it is achieved.

   ii   What are the generally accepted reasons or indications for advising coronary artery bypass surgery?

23   Coronary artery bypass surgery is said to improve the prognosis (i.e. reduce the mortality) of angina with stenosis of certain coronary arteries. Which are they? Up to what age is coronary artery surgery performed? What are the pros and cons of coronary artery bypass in patients with poor left ventricular function?

24   What degree of stenosis of a coronary artery is usually required before coronary artery bypass surgery is recommended?

25   Which is a greater threat to life, a proximal or a distal stenosis of a coronary artery?

26   What in percentage terms is the likelihood of coronary artery bypass surgery relieving angina?

27   What in percentage terms is the mortality of coronary artery bypass surgery?

28   What in percentage terms is the likelihood of restenosis 10 years after coronary artery bypass surgery?

29   What is balloon angioplasty? What does it do to the arterial wall? In which patients is it currently indicated? What are its main disadvantages?

Answers

21   Coronary arteriography

Arteriography involves demonstrating the anatomy of an artery by the injection of opaque contrast medium along its course. In the case of coronary arteriography this is through a catheter introduced into a coronary ostium via the femoral or brachial artery.

Indications

●   Coronary angiography is indicated in those cases in which coronary artery bypass surgery or angioplasty is contemplated.

●   Occasionally coronary arteriography is also performed for diagnostic reasons to assess the severity of disease in patients with severe symptoms but in whom there are doubts about the diagnosis after clinical assessment and exercise testing.

22   Coronary artery bypass surgery

i   Coronary artery bypass surgery involves bypassing an atheromatous obstruction in a coronary artery by one of three methods:

●   Taking a vein from the leg, reversing it because of the valves, and suturing one end to the aorta and the other to the coronary artery distal to the obstruction.

●   Inserting the internal mammary artery into the left anterior descending artery distal to the obstruction.

●   Endarterectomy, that is direct removal of an atheromatous obstruction.

ii   There are two main indications for coronary artery bypass surgery:

●   Relief of angina not controlled by medical treatment.

●   Improvement of the prognosis.

In addition, adult patients undergoing heart valve surgery may also have coronary artery bypass surgery if there is significant coexisting disease of the coronary arteries.

23   Prognosis and the vessels involved

Several trials have been conducted to compare the effect on prognosis of surgical versus medical treatment of angina. However, because of failure to randomly enter all eligible patients into these trials their results are inconclusive. Nonetheless, at the present time it seems that coronary artery bypass surgery improves the prognosis where there is significant stenosis of:

●   The main stem of the left coronary artery.

●   Two vessels but only if one is the left anterior descending artery.

●   Three or more vessels.

●   In addition, although unproven at the present time by randomised trial, coronary artery bypass surgery may improve the prognosis in patients with:

a   unstable or continuous angina at rest

b   patients with angina or ECG evidence of ischaemia after myocardial infarction.

NOTE: The prognosis of one vessel disease is similar with either surgical or medical treatment.

●   Age of the patient. Because their expectation of active life should be longer the indication for surgery is relatively stronger in young persons. The upper age for coronary artery bypass is generally agreed to be the early or middle seventies, although coronary artery bypass has been carried out successfully in many otherwise fit patients in their eighties with angina disrupting their life style despite full medical treatment.

●   Poor function of the left ventricle. Operation is contraindicated in patients with frank left ventricular failure,

a   because the risks of surgery in this group of patients are increased, and b   because operation does not improve the function of previously damaged myocardium.

However, coronary artery bypass has been found to improve the prognosis of patients with angina severe enough to justify operation, who are not in cardiac failure, but have a very low ejection fraction, for instance as low as 30%.

24   Significant stenosis of a coronary artery

It is generally agreed that surgery is indicated only in cases where there is marked stenosis with occlusion > 70% of a vessel's lumen.

25   Threat to life and proximal versus distal stenosis

Because it threatens a larger amount of myocardium, a proximal lesion is a more serious threat to life than a distal lesion.

26   The likelihood of coronary artery surgery relieving angina

Substantial relief is achieved in about 80%.

27   The mortality of coronary artery surgery

With an experienced surgical team, in otherwise fit persons with normal or near normal left ventricular function, the mortality of the operation is about 1%. As implied above, the mortality is increased in those with poor left ventricular function.

28   The likelihood of restenosis over 10 years

Restenosis occurs in about 5% of grafts per year. Thus after about 10 years 50% of grafts have restenosed.

29   Balloon angioplasty

This involves dilatation of a stenosed artery by passing a balloon catheter into the stenosis and inflating the balloon to a predetermined size under controlled pressure. The mechanism by which dilatation is produced is by stretching the vessel, cracking the media and intima, and possibly also by compression of soft plaques. The technique is suitable for proximal lesions of the coronary arteries. The indications for balloon angioplasty are increasing. Currently the indications are angina with one vessel disease not responding to medical treatment, and angina not responding to medical treatment in patients with multivessel disease who are not fit to undergo coronary artery surgery.

The disadvantages of balloon angioplasty are that in a few cases emergency coronary artery bypass surgery becomes necessary during the procedure, and that in about 25% of cases restenosis of the artery and angina occur within a few months.

Further Reading

Braunwald E (ed) (1984). *Heart Disease*, 2nd edition. WB
    Saunders, Philadelphia. Chapters 8, exercise stress testing; 10,
    coronary arteriography; 11, radioisotope examination; 38,
    chronic coronary artery disease.

Coronary Artery Surgery Study (CASS) (1983). A randomized trial
    of coronary artery bipass surgery survival data. *Circulation 68*,
    939-50.

European Coronary Surgery Study Group (1982). Longterm results
    of prospective randomized study of coronary artery surgery in
    stable angina pectoris. *Lancet ii*, 1173-80.

Hampton JR (1986). *The ECG Made Easy*, 3rd edition. Churchill
    Livingstone, Edinburgh.

Ross R (1986)). The pathogenesis of atherosclerosis—an update.
    N.Engl.J.Med. 314, 488-500.

Case D
A Case of Chest Pain — No. 2: Mrs C-B, aged 65 years

A happily married housewife living with her husband in their own modern semi-detached house.

History of present condition

Whilst digging in the garden on a sunny afternoon this lady suddenly developed severe tight pain across the chest, radiating to the left arm and through to the back. The pain was accompanied by profuse sweating and a profound feeling of weakness, and continued for 3 hours despite an injection of morphine 10 mg intramuscularly given by her family doctor, and a second similar injection on admission to hospital.

There was no previous history of chest pain, but the patient volunteered that she experienced pain in the right calf after walking approximately a quarter of a mile.

Past medical history

Hysterectomy 30 years previously, for reasons of which she was not clear.
No past history of hypertension or diabetes.

Relevant direct questions

Breathlessness: nil.
Swelling of ankles: nil.
Medications: nil.
Smoking: 20 cigarettes per day since adolescence.
Alcoholic intake: 6–8 alcoholic drinks at weekends.

Examination

Pale sweaty ill looking middle-aged lady with lined, pinched smoker's face and nicotine stained fingers, lying quietly because of pain in the chest.

Cardiovascular system

No breathlessness, cyanosis, splinter haemorrhages or finger clubbing.
Pulse 90 regular, moderate volume.
BP90/60 lying.
Jugular venous pulse (JVP) not raised.
Apex impalpable.

Right ventricle not heaving.
Heart sounds very quiet—almost inaudible.
No audible added sounds or murmurs.

Other systems

Examination of the other systems was normal except for bilateral late crackles at the bases of the lung fields, and absence of the dorsalis pedis and posterior tibial pulses in the right foot (both pulses were present on the left).

Comment on the history

●   This case illustrates the importance of making introductory statements about the general condition of the patient at the beginning of the examination notes. Such a statement should convey an overall picture of the patient with particular reference to any appearance of being well or unwell. It is surprising how often this is omitted. In the present instance the details taken from the notes tell us that:
a   the patient was sweaty, unwell and lying quietly because of pain in the chest, and,
b   she smoked.
●   The examination also revealed absence of the foot pulses on the right. Being an effective clinician is very much a matter of discipline, and it is an important part of the discipline of the examination of all new patients to *routinely* examine the foot pulses, just as it is important to *routinely* listen for carotid and renal bruits, examine the fundi, the limb reflexes, and when indicated, the sensory system.

Further history

On the day following her initial chest pain Mrs C-B had further pain across the chest lasting half an hour. This was associated with episodes lasting 5 minutes of sinus bradycardia, complete heart block, and then a short period of atrial flutter and Wenckebach phenomenon. Thereafter sinus rhythm was maintained. There were no changes in the examination of the patient, and subsequently she made an uneventful recovery from her illness and was discharged home.

Mrs C-B

Questions

1   What diagnosis is suggested by the history and physical findings?
2   What are the two specific investigations performed in ordinary clinical practice to confirm or refute the suggested diagnosis?
3   Why do you think the heart sounds were quiet in this case?
4   What does the blood pressure reading and the presence of bilateral basal crackles suggest?

5   What was the pain in the right calf due to? Taken in the total context of the case, what does it imply?

6   What do you think may have happened to Mrs C-B when she had further chest pain and arrhythmias on her second day in hospital? How might the episode have been investigated?

7   Mrs C-B experienced several arrhythmias including sinus bradycardia and complete heart block. At which site is a myocardial infarct most likely to be associated with these arrhythmias? What is the explanation of this?

Answers

1   The diagnosis suggested by Mrs C-B's chest pain

The history of tight substernal chest pain radiating to the left arm, accompanied by sweating and a feeling of prostration, all lasting for several hours despite rest, suggested that until proved otherwise the patient had suffered a myocardial infarction.

The diagnosis was supported by the findings of quiet heart sounds, low blood pressure and crackles at the lung bases.

2   The specific investigations used in ordinary clinical practice to confirm or refute a diagnosis of myocardial infarction

● The electrocardiograph (ECG)—the changes associated with myocardial infarction are described on page 118.

● Measurement of the serum enzymes, discussed on page 121.

3   Mrs C-B's quiet heart sounds

The causes of quiet heart sounds are discussed on page 18. In Mrs C-B's case they were caused by her myocardial infarction. In this condition the heart sounds may be of normal intensity, although in many cases they are *muffled, quiet or distant* due to *decreased velocity of closure of the valves* resulting from impaired contraction of the damaged ventricular muscle.

4   The significance of Mrs C-B's low blood pressure and bilateral basal crackles

These suggest left ventricular failure. The low blood pressure suggests 'forward' failure, and the basal crackles 'backward' failure. An explanation of the concepts of forward and backward failure is given on page 32.

5   The cause of the pain in Mrs C-B's right calf

Pain in the calf that comes *immediately* on walking may be due to *acute* conditions such as a torn muscle or ligament, superficial thrombophlebitis or deep vein thrombosis. *Chronic* pain that *comes after walking a certain distance*, especially as in this case, when accompanied by absence of the foot pulses, is usually due to atherosclerosis causing arterial insufficiency—a condition known as *intermittent claudication* from the Latin *claudus* meaning lame.

Taken in conjunction with her myocardial infarction it suggests that Mrs C-B was suffering from widespread atherosclerosis—that she was an *arteriopath*.

6   Mrs C-B's further chest pain and arrhythmias

This suggested that she may have extended her original myocardial infarct or suffered a new infarction at another site. This occurs in up to about 5% of cases, and may be investigated by repeating the ECG to see if there are further changes, and also by repeating measurement of the serum enzymes. Subject to the limitations discussed on page 122, a second rise in the serum enzymes, especially when associated with a history of further typical chest pain or ECG changes, is highly suggestive of reinfarction.

7   The site of myocardial infarction most likely to be associated with sinus bradycardia and complete heart block

Sinus bradycardia and complete heart block occur much more frequently with an inferior infarct (ECG leads II, III and aVf) than with an anterior infarct (ECG leads V_1–V_6). This is because in about 85% of persons the blood supply to the S-A and A-V nodes comes from branches of the right coronary artery which also supplies the inferior border of the heart. Very large anterior infarcts extending backwards into the interventricular septum to involve the conducting tissue may also cause complete heart block, and because of their large size carry a poor prognosis.

Chapter 6
Myocardial Infarction

Definition; risk factors; mortality

Questions

1   Define the term 'myocardial infarction'.

2   List and make comments on the risk factors such as hypercholesterolaemia associated with death from ischaemic heart disease. Also list and make comments on the factors thought to protect against ischaemic heart disease.

3   Which factors in cigarette smoke are thought to be responsible for (i) accelerated atherosclerosis, (ii) sudden death, (iii) carcinoma of the lung, and (iv) the addictive and psychological effects of smoking?

4   What is the percentage likelihood of a patient with a myocardial infarction having a past history of angina, myocardial infarction, or hypertension?

5i   What is the percentage of patients with acute myocardial infarction dying: before reaching hospital; in hospital; in the first year after discharge from hospital?

ii   Out of the total number of patients who die, what percentage of the deaths occur within the first two hours of the onset of symptoms? Why is this so important? Among the survivors, what is the age adjusted mortality after 10 years?

Answers

1   Definition

Myocardial infarction is defined as death of cardiac muscle due to a sudden reduction of the blood supply along a coronary artery as a result of thrombosis, atheromatous narrowing, or a combination of the two, or an embolus.

2   The main risk factors for death from ischaemic heart disease, and protective factors

Risk factors

●   *Increasing age*. The incidence of death from ischaemic heart disease increases by decade up to the age of about 85 years.

●   *Male sex*. Prior to the menopause, clinical ischaemic heart disease is rare in women, and until aged about 70 is commoner in males than females.

●   *Hyperlipidaemia*. Many studies comparing populations in different countries have led to the appreciation of a direct relationship between the mean serum cholesterol of a population, low density lipoproteins (on which most of the cholesterol in the plasma is carried) and the incidence of death from ischaemic heart disease. By contrast, the role of plasma triglycerides and very low density lipoproteins (on which most of the triglycerides are carried) in the pathogenesis of ischaemic heart disease is unclear.

Apart from the direct relationship between the mean level of serum cholesterol within a population and risk of dying from ischaemic heart disease, it also appears that other risk factors such as hypertension and smoking are probably effective only if the mean serum cholesterol of the population is elevated.

The level of serum cholesterol and of the lipoproteins is determined by both *genetic factors* such as indigenous production and degradation, and *environmental factors* such as the amount of fat in the diet. Studies of populations in different countries show that the intake of polysaturated fat in the diet is the most important factor determining the serum cholesterol and mortality from ischaemic heart disease within a population. Thus the type of fat eaten appears to be more important than the quantity. Whereas polysaturated fats of the type eaten in Britain and Finland cause serum cholesterol and low density lipoproteins to rise, monounsaturated fats, such as olive oil eaten in Italy and Spain, probably cause the serum cholesterol to fall. In part this may explain the different incidence of ischaemic heart disease in the various countries. Reducing dietary intake of cholesterol and saturated fats reduces plasma lipids by about 10-20% on average, and although unproven in a large population, hopefully reduces mortality from ischaemic heart disease.

• *Hypertension*. In men aged less than 45 years, the risk of death from ischaemic heart disease is related more to elevation of diastolic than systolic blood pressure, and in men aged over 60 more to elevation of systolic pressure. In men aged 45-60 years the risk is approximately the same for elevation of either pressure.

Although the treatment of hypertension reduces the incidence of stroke, heart failure and renal failure, it has only a marginal effect on the mortality of myocardial infarction.

• *Smoking*. There is a linear relationship between the number of cigarettes smoked per day and the risk of dying of ischaemic heart disease. The factors in cigarette smoke responsible for this are discussed in the answer to question 3.

• *Pre-existing evidence of ischaemic heart disease*. Either clinical angina or ECG evidence of ischaemia are risk factors for death from ischaemic heart disease.

• *Family history of ischaemic heart disease*. This factor results from the familial tendency to hyperlipidaemia, hypertension and diabetes, although in some families unrecognised factors operate.

• *Diabetes*. Due to the micro- and macrovascular disease with which diabetes is associated, the occurrence and mortality of ischaemic heart disease among diabetics is more than twice that of non-diabetics.

- *Obesity*. Because of confounding factors such as hyperlipidaemia and hypertension, both of which are associated with obesity, opinion is divided about the contribution obesity makes to the incidence of death from ischaemic heart disease. However, it is now recognised that abdominal obesity, giving the person an 'apple' shape, indicated by an increased ratio of abdominal/hip girth is an independent risk factor, whereas obesity around the buttocks and thighs, giving the person a 'pear' shape, is not.
- *Personality*. It has been suggested, but is disputed, that on the basis of their personalities the population can be divided into two groups at differing risk of death from ischaemic heart disease. According to this hypothesis group A are those persons at risk because of intense competitiveness, easily provoked hostility and a sense of being under time pressure, whilst group B, at lesser risk, are those persons with more contented or placid personalities who nonetheless may be very able achievers.
- *Above average levels of blood clotting factors*. Traditionally death from ischaemic heart disease has been associated with atherosclerosis in the vessel wall. Recently, however, attention has focused on hypercoagulability of the blood as an important risk factor. Raised levels of fibrinogen, in part due to smoking, raised levels of factor VII, due mainly to dietary fat, and of factor VIII and an inhibitor of plasminogen activity (PAI) are now each recognised as risk factors for intra-arterial thrombosis and death from ischaemic heart disease.

Protective factors

- *Physical activity*. There have been several large studies involving thousands of subjects showing the protective effect of *regular* physical exercise in middle-aged men. It has been suggested that the minimum requirement is probably about 20 minutes $\times$ 3 per week, raising the pulse to more than 130 beats per minute.
- *High density lipoprotein (HDL)*. This lipoprotein is thought to carry cholesterol away from the arterial wall to the liver (unlike low density lipoprotein which is associated with its deposition) and therefore to protect against the development of atherosclerosis. Most epidemiological surveys support this view although one large recent survey suggests that when smoking and obesity are allowed for high density lipoprotein is not cardioprotective.
- *Diet*. Eating a diet low in fat lowers the incidence of ischaemic heart disease in those with very high serum levels of cholesterol. Screening for such individuals is therefore indicated. However, as yet it is unproven that lowering the fat intake of the *whole* population, most of whom have a normal serum cholesterol, will have a greatly added protective effect. Nonetheless current recommendations to lower the fat content of the diet from about 40% of total calories to about 30% seem prudent.

- *Prophylactic aspirin.* Although regular prophylactic aspirin has a beneficial effect in persons who have had a heart attack, the two published trials of regular aspirin prophylaxis in *healthy* middle-aged men (doctors in fact) have produced different results making it difficult to know whether regular aspirin prophylaxis is indicated in the healthy middle-aged, although it is possible that it may be.

3 Smoking

This is associated with accelerated atherosclerosis and increased mortality from ischaemic heart disease, particularly of sudden death. The factors responsible for the effects of smoking are as follows:

i   *Accelerated atherosclerosis* is probably due to a multiplicity of substances within tobacco smoke rather than a single substance.

ii   *Sudden death*, on the other hand, is probably due to carbon monoxide predisposing to arrhythmias as a result of reduction of the oxygen content of the blood and increased levels of carboxy-haemoglobin. Because these changes are rapidly reversible, not surprisingly this risk is rapidly reduced in those who stop smoking.

iii   *Carcinoma of the lung* is probably due to the tars within tobacco smoke.

iv   *The addictive and psychological effects* of smoking are thought to be due to nicotine mimicking acetylcholine in the brain and in the sympathetic and parasympathetic ganglia. The result is complex. Depending upon the smoker's environment, nicotine has either stimulating or depressing effects.

4   The likelihood of a history of previous cardiovascular disease in a case of myocardial infarction

- Previous angina: 40%
- Previous myocardial infarction: 20%
- Previous hypertension: 20%

5   Deaths from acute myocardial infarction

i   The percentage of patients with acute myocardial infarction dying:
- Before reaching hospital: 25%
- In hospital: 10–15%
- During the first year after hospitalisation: 10%

ii   Half the deaths occur within the first 2 hours of the onset of infarction. Efforts to minimise mortality therefore need to be concentrated on this crucial very short period.

Even after 10 years, the age adjusted mortality is three and a half times normal.

Symptoms and signs; clinical monitoring
Questions

6   List the various ways in which myocardial infarction may present, and add a note about the underlying mechanism of each. What percentage of myocardial infarctions are painless?

7   List and write a line or two explaining the main signs found in patients with myocardial infarction.

8   Patients who have a myocardial infarct need to be properly observed. What clinical parameters would you monitor, that is what clinical observations would you make yourself and ask the nurses to make in the coronary care unit (CCU) in the routine management of a patient following a myocardial infarct?

Answers

6   Presentation

Myocardial infarction may present in any of the following ways:

● *Death*: 50% occur within the first 2 hours. In the majority of cases death shortly after the onset of symptoms is due to ventricular fibrillation, although following a large infarct death may occur as a result of failure of the pumping action of the heart.

● *Chest pain* occurs in 80–85% of cases. In the remaining 15–20% infarction is painless, particularly among those who are diabetic and elderly. Typically the pain of infarction occurs at rest or persists despite rest after exertion. Usually it is more severe than any previous angina, being described as a tight, squeezing or crushing pain across the chest, radiating in two-thirds of cases to the arms, neck or jaw. Due to autonomic upset, nausea, vomiting and sweating may occur.

● *Loss of consciousness* may occur due either to an arrhythmia, or to left ventricular dysfunction, particularly if the latter is a result of involvement of the main stem of the left coronary artery.

● *Breathlessness* may be present as a result of left ventricular failure.

● *Sudden 'unwellness' or weakness* may also occur as a result of left ventricular dysfunction and autonomic upset.

7   Signs

● *General appearance.* This may be normal, or the patient may look very ill, or as a result of pain may appear frightened, anxious, sweaty or restless. If the circulation is impaired the periphery may be cold and cyanosed.

● *Pyrexia* may develop during the first 48 hours and is due to tissue necrosis.

● *The pulse* is usually regular, but may be irregular if there is an arrhythmia, or weak if the pumping action of the heart is greatly impaired.

● *The heart sounds* may be of normal intensity, or quiet or muffled (see page 18). Due to lack of compliance and stiffness of the ventricles added sounds may be audible. The mechanisms underlying these are explained on page 20. A fourth heart sound is usually audible. A third heart sound generally reflects a large infarct and cardiac dilatation.

● *A murmur of mitral regurgitation* may be heard and indicates dysfunction or rupture of a papillary muscle. Most commonly this occurs with an inferior infarct involving the posterior cusp of the mitral valve.

● *A pericardial rub* occurring within the first day or so of the illness indicates a full thickness or transmural infarct causing inflammation of the pericardium. A rub occurring after a week or so is suggestive of Dressler's syndrome (see page 146).

● *The blood pressure* may be *normal*, or *low* if there is failure of the pumping action of the left ventricle, or *high* if the patient is in *pain* or is hypertensive.

● *Heart failure* may occur. Usually this is left ventricular. However, right ventricular failure can occur as a result of left ventricular failure, or as a result of infarction of part of the right ventricle as happens in up to about 30% of inferior infarcts.

8   The clinical parameters that should be monitored

Assessing a patient as a whole person is the essence of good care in every situation, but nowhere is this more important than in the coronary care or intensive care units. Each time a patient is seen the following should be assessed automatically:

General appearance of the patient

Whether they look well or ill, their colour, whether they are anxious, in pain, breathless, or cyanosed.

Routine clinical measurements

● Temperature.
● Respiratory rate.
● Pulse and blood pressure.
● Central venous pressure (CVP) if it is being monitored.
● Fluid balance. Fluid intake and urinary output. It is particularly important to monitor urinary output as it reflects perfusion of the kidneys.
● ECG and cardiac monitor. Being able to identify ventricular arrhythmias as they occur is part of the raison d'être of the coronary care unit.

Specific examinaion of the cardiorespiratory system

● Quality and rhythm of the pulse.
● Jugular venous pulse (JVP).
● Palpation to assess the position of the cardiac apex.
● Palpation of the sternum to assess right ventricular heave.

● Auscultation for added sounds (i.e. III or IV sounds), new murmurs, pericardial rub.
● Examination of the lung bases to assess whether there is dullness to percussion reflecting effusion or collapse, or crackles reflecting pulmonary oedema, infection or pulmonary infarction.
● Examination of the sacrum to assess whether there is oedema reflecting cardiac failure.
● Examination of the legs to assess whether there is oedema suggestive of cardiac failure or calf tenderness suggestive of deep vein thrombosis (DVT). In order to avoid the latter, patients should be encouraged to move and not cross their legs.

Investigation (i)
Questions

9 Upon what triad of symptoms and investigations is the diagnosis of myocardial infarction usually based?
10 What basic laboratory investigations would you order in a case of myocardial infarction?
11i Describe the typical sequence of ECG changes seen during the evolution of a full thickness myocardial infarct. What are the changes of subendocardial or partial thickness infarction, and of posterior infarction?
ii In which ECG leads are infarcts in the following areas seen: anteroseptal, anterior, anterolateral, inferior, posterior?

Answers

9 The triad of symptoms and investigations used in the diagnosis of myocardial infarction

The convention is that two of the following should be present:
● *A history of typical chest pain.*
● *Typical or appropriate ECG changes.* The most specific change is the development of Q waves, although other changes such as the development of a raised ST segment or arrow-head symmetrical T wave inversion may be used in the presence of enzyme changes.
● *Elevation of the appropriate serum enzymes* to twice normal levels.

10 Basic laboratory investigations

● *Full blood count.* A neutrophilia or polymorphonuclear leucocytosis, typically up to 12–15 000, may occur and is a non-specific marker of tissue necrosis.
● *Erythrocyte sedimentation rate (ESR).* Elevation may occur during the first one or two weeks and is a non-specific marker of tissue necrosis.
● *ECG.* Discussed in the answer to question 11.
● *Measurement of serum enzymes.* Discussed in the answers to questions 12 and 13.

●   *Measurement of serum urea and electrolytes* to check renal function, and also to check for hypokalaemia.
●   *Chest x-ray*. Chiefly to check for evidence of heart failure or pulmonary embolus.

11i   The typical sequence of ECG changes during the evolution of a myocardial infarct

Several combinations of changes may occur in the QRS complex, the ST segment or the T wave, but the typical sequence of changes is as follows:
●   *Within hours* the development of a raised ST segment. This is the so-called 'current of injury', and is due to failure of the ST

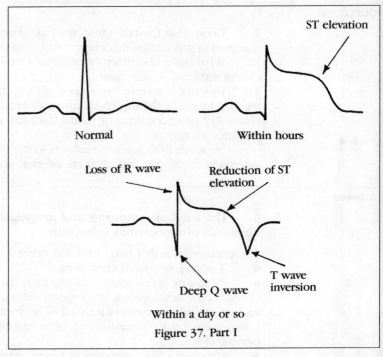

Figure 37. Part I

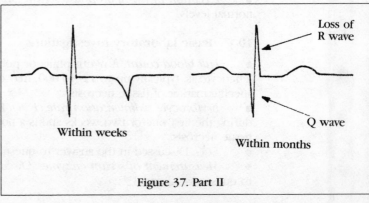

Figure 37. Part II

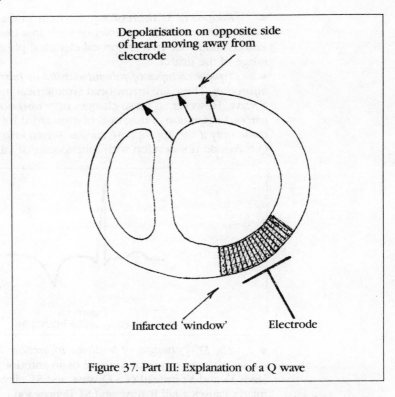

Figure 37. Part III: Explanation of a Q wave

segment to return to the isoelectric point as a result of *incomplete repolarisation of the damaged myocardium* relative to the surrounding normal tissue.

●　　*Within 1-3 days: reduction in the height of the R wave.* The size of the R wave is a reflection of left ventricular muscle mass. As a consequence it becomes smaller when the muscle mass is reduced by infarction.

●　　*Development of a deep Q wave.* Three aspects are important here:

a　　Q waves are caused by the infarcted area of ventricle under the electrode being unable to produce a large R wave. The electrode therefore picks up the depolarisation of the opposite side of the heart as it travels out from the endocardium to the epicardium, that is away from the electrode. This results in a negative or down wave, that is a Q or QS wave.

b　　Q waves are considered to be significant if they are 25% of the R wave that follows them.

c　　Q waves may persist for years as a marker of a previous infarct. However, it is important to remember that they may occur with cardiomyopathies and tumours of the heart.

●　　*Gradual reduction of ST elevation* occurs with the development of arrow-head symmetrical T wave inversion due to abnormalities of repolarisation. Persistence of ST elevation reflects a dyskinetic area of myocardium and should alert the attending doctor to the possibility of a cardiac aneurysm.

• *Reciprocal ST depression* may occur in the leads opposite an infarct, for example in the inferior leads in a case of an anterior infarct, and is due to a reciprocal electrical phenomenon or mirror image of the infarct.

• *Typical changes of subendocardial or partial thickness infarction.* These are arrow-head symmetrical inversion of the T wave. However, as these changes *may also occur with ischaemia without infarction*, a diagnosis of myocardial infarction should be made only if the appropriate cardiac serum enzymes are elevated. Q waves do not develop with subendocardial infarction.

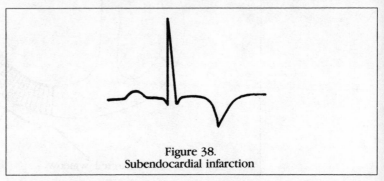

Figure 38.
Subendocardial infarction

• *The ECG changes of posterior infarction.* A posterior infarct causes changes opposite to those of an anterior infarct. Thus in leads V1 and V2 instead of a Q wave and ST elevation, a posterior infarct causes a tall R wave and ST depression or an upright T wave. The cause of the tall R wave in leads V1 and V2 is demonstrated in Figure 39.

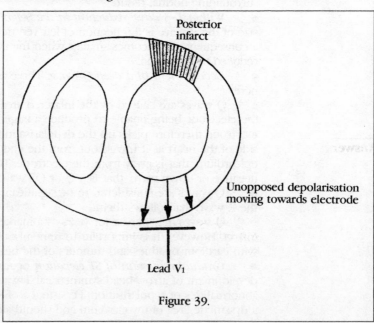

Posterior infarct

Unopposed depolarisation moving towards electrode

Lead V1

Figure 39.

Because the infarcted back of the heart is electrically inactive the electrode picks up only the depolarisation from the front of the heart as it travels out from the endocardium to the epicardium. The result of the impulse travelling towards the electrode is to produce a positive wave, that is an R wave. Posterior infarction is usually associated with inferior infarction.

NOTE: Infarction of the right ventricle may occur but the ECG changes associated with it are non-specific. Because the artery to the right ventricle is a branch of the right coronary artery, infarction of the right ventricle is usually associated with inferior infarction of the left ventricle.

11ii   ECG leads and site of infarction

This is fully disussed on page 91, and may be summarised as follows:

Site of infarction	ECG leads
● Anteroseptal	V_1–V_3
● Anterior	V_1–V_6
● Anterolateral	V_4–V_6, I and aVl
● Inferior	II, III, aVf
● Posterior	V_1 and V_2

Investigation (ii): enzyme measurement
Questions

12   Which enzymes are commonly measured in the diagnosis of myocardial infarction? At what times after the infarct does each of them typically peak? What rise is generally accepted as diagnostic?

13i   Which is the most cardiospecific enzyme in the diagnosis of myocardial infarction?

ii   Apart from the heart, from which other organs may aspartate transaminase (AST) be released?

iii   In what conditions other than myocardial infarction may elevated levels of serum enzymes be encountered?

iv   Might an intramuscular injection or DC shock to the heart affect the levels of the serum enzymes?

Answers

12   Enzyme measurement

The enzymes most commonly measured in the diagnosis of myocardial infarction are listed below. It is important to take blood for their measurement at the times after the onset of symptoms at which they most typically peak. It is generally agreed that a rise to twice normal levels is necessary for a positive diagnosis.

● Aspartate transaminase (AST), also known as serum glutamic oxaloacetic transaminase (SGOT) About 24-48 hours
● Creatine kinase (total) (CK) About 24 hours
● Creatine kinase–MB isoenzyme (CK–MB) About 24 hours
● Lactic dehydrogenase isoenzyme-1 (LDH), also known as hydroxybutyric dehydrogenase (HBD) About 3-4 days

NOTE: Five isoenzymes of lactic dehydrogenase are recognised. Heart muscle contains more of the isoenzyme LDH-1 than liver or skeletal muscle which is the reason it is preferred to the other isoenzymes of LDH in the diagnosis of myocardial infarction.

13   Serum enzymes, the heart and other organs

i   The most cardiospecific serum enzyme is the isoenzyme CK–MB. This is because the heart is the only organ to contain it in large amounts. Small amounts are contained in tissues such as skeletal muscle, but raised levels due to this are found only with widespread and extensive damage of skeletal muscle such as occurs in muscular dystrophy or crush injury.

ii   Aspartate transaminase is contained in many tissues and organs including lung, liver, pancreas, gut, kidney and red blood cells. Raised levels of this enzyme are therefore a non-specific marker of tissue damage.

iii   With the exception of CK–MB, serum levels of the most commonly measured enzymes may be elevated in conditions such as pulmonary infarction, hepatic congestion due to right heart failure, liver diseases such as hepatitis, acute pancreatitis, intestinal and renal infarction, muscular diseases such as dermatomyositis and muscular dystrophy, and haemolytic anaemia.

iv   It has been shown that an intramuscular injection may cause elevation of total CK. Because of the trauma it causes to the muscles of the chest wall, DC shock generally causes elevation of the serum enzymes, although any effect on CK–MB is usually small.

All these changes may lead to confusion when injections are given or myocardial infarction is complicated by pulmonary embolus, hepatic congestion due to right heart failure, or administered DC shock.

Immediate treatment
Questions

14   List the main aims of the treatment of myocardial infarction.
15   What are the advantages and disadvantages of hospital coronary care units? Which patients might be treated at home, and which should be treated in a coronary care unit after a myocardial infarct?
16   What are the names, doses and routes of administration of the drugs most commonly used for analgesia after myocardial

infarction? What are their main side effects?

17   What is the purpose of rest after myocardial infarction?

18   List the drugs whose immediate prophylactic use reduces the mortality of myocardial infarction. What is the rationale behind the use of each drug?

19   What, if any, are the indications for anticoagulants following myocardial infarction?

Answers

14   The aims of treatment

- Relief of pain
- Limitation of infarct size
- Treatment of complications
- Prevention of further infarction

15   The advantages and disadvantages of coronary care units and home versus hospital treatment

The advantages

- The justification of the CCU is that by making it possible to continuously monitor the ECG it provides the facility for the immediate detection and treatment of life threatening ventricular arrhythmias, principally ventricular fibrillation, which is fatal within minutes unless treated.
- Facilities are also available for the administration of drugs that reduce the acute mortality of myocardial infarction, and allow the immediate treatment of complications such as heart failure or shock, or conditions requiring intubation, ventilation or cardiac pacing.

The disadvantages

- The fear that may be engendered by the unnatural surroundings and high technology.
- The fear that may be engendered by the death of other patients on the unit.

It is possible, but not proven, that the fear may stimulate the sympathetic nervous system to cause arrhythmias, or as a result of sinus tachycardia increase the oxygen consumption of the heart and cause the infarct to extend.

Against this background the following guidelines would seem appropriate.

Patients who probably may be treated safely at home

Those seen at home 12 or more hours after the onset of symptoms so long as they appear well, are no longer in pain and show no evidence of arrhythmia or heart failure.

Patients who should be transferred to CCU

Those seen within a few hours of the onset of symptoms, or those with continuing pain or symptoms or signs suggestive of complications.

16   The drugs used for analgesia after myocardial infarction

Many drugs are recommended, but the two most commonly used are morphine and diamorphine (heroin). Weight for weight, diamorphine is about twice as potent as morphine. The doses of each are therefore:
- Morphine, 5–10 mg intravenously for quick action, or 10–20 mg intramuscularly.
- Diamorphine, 5 mg intravenously for quick action, or 5–10 mg intramuscularly.

The main side effects of both drugs are:
- *Nausea and vomiting* due to stimulation of the brain stem. Because of this it is usual to give an antiemetic such as metoclopramide 10 mg or perphenazine 5 mg with the opiate.
- *Respiratory depression* due to depression of the respiratory centre. Because of this opiates should be either withheld or given very cautiously in reduced dosage to chronic bronchitics of the blue bloating type.
- *Hypotension* may occur as a result of relaxation of venous vascular smooth muscle.

17   The purpose of rest after myocardial infarction

Rest is recommended during the first day or so in an effort to minimise the work of the heart and the oxygen requirements of any ischaemic muscle around the infarct in the hope of (a) limiting the size of the infarct, and (b) minimising the risk of arrhythmia.

18   Drugs that reduce the mortality of myocardial infarction

Given intravenously (orally in the case of aspirin) within a few hours of the onset of symptoms each of the following drugs reduces the mortality of myocardial infarction by about 1–3 patients for every 100 patients treated:
- Beta blocking drugs
- Streptokinase
- Tissue plasminogen activator
- Aspirin

- *Beta blockers*. These drugs reduce the *acute* mortality of myocardial infarction by about one in 200 patients and prevent cardiac arrest in one, and reinfarction in another. The reduction in mortality is probably due to a reduction in the incidence of rupture of the softened area of the infarct. Presumably this is a result of the negative inotropic action of the drug reducing the power of contraction of the heart muscle.

- *Streptokinase*. Thrombosis within a coronary artery is thought to occur in about 80% of myocardial infarcts. Streptokinase digests fibrin, fibrinogen, prothrombin and clotting factors V and VII throughout the circulation. The rationale of using streptokinase is to lyse the thrombus as soon as possible after the onset of symptoms so as to restore the circulation sufficiently to prevent the infarction of ischaemic areas around the infarct. Used in this way streptokinase reduces the mortality of myocardial infarction by about 2-3 patients for every 100 patients treated.
- *Tissue plasminogen activator*. The rationale of using this drug is similar to that of streptokinase except that whereas streptokinase causes generalised fibrinolysis, tissue plasminogen activator acts more specifically upon the clot. It is reported that tissue plasminogen activator reduces the mortality of myocardial infarction by about three patients for every 100 patients treated.
- *Aspirin*. The rationale behind the use of aspirin is to inhibit platelet aggregation by inhibiting the production of thromboxane A_2. This is discussed on page 232. Given to patients with myocardial infarction aspirin is reported to save the lives of 2-3 patients for every 100 patients treated.
- *Streptokinase plus aspirin*. Compared with the use of each alone, in combination these drugs have an added effect reducing the mortality of myocardial infarction by a further 1-2 patients for every 100 treated.

19 The indications, if any, for anticoagulants after myocardial infarction

Neither heparin nor warfarin lyses coronary thrombi. However, they do reduce the incidence of arterial and venous thromboembolism. Anticoagulants are therefore indicated, usually during the hospital stay only, for patients at an increased risk of these complications, that is patients who are clinically ill, in heart failure or shock, or for patients with varicose veins or a past history of deep vein thrombosis or pulmonary embolism.

Complications
Questions

20   List and write short notes about the clinical features and treatment of the complications of myocardial infarction.
21   Are ventricular extrasystoles of prognostic importance in the hours or days immediately after myocardial infarction?
22   Give two possible reasons why patients may develop sinus tachycardia after myocardial infarction. Would you treat it?
23   What effect is the onset of atrial fibrillation shortly after the beginning of the illness likely to have upon the prognosis of myocardial infarction? How would you treat it? In what situation would you cardiovert the patient using DC shock?
24   What are the indications for treating sinus bradycardia after myocardial infarction? How is it treated?

25 What are the indications for a temporary pacemaker after myocardial infarction?

Answers

20 The complications of myocardial infarction

- *Death*. Details of the interval between the onset of symptoms and the likelihood of death are discussed on page 114.
- *Heart failure*. Full details of the pathogenesis, symptoms and signs of heart failure are given on page 27 onwards.
- *Arrhythmia*. Supraventricular arrhythmias are discussed on page 63, and ventricular arrhythmias on page 72.
- *Heart block*. This is discussed on page 55.
- *Cardiogenic shock*. This is discussed on page 130.
- *Pulmonary embolus*. These arise from leg or pelvic veins and are an indication for immediate treatment with heparin.
- *Arterial embolus*. These arise from thrombus that has formed on the inflamed endocardium, and may cause a stroke or ischaemia or gangrene of the leg, or infarction of a kidney or piece of gut. In an effort to prevent further emboli, immediate anticoagulation with heparin is indicated at the first hint of an arterial embolus. Immediate embolectomy will usually save a leg. Infarcted bowel must be resected.
- *Pericarditis*. This is discussed on page 143.
- *Mitral regurgitation*. This is signalled by the development of an apical systolic murmur radiating to the axilla and is usually a result of stretching or rupture of a papillary muscle in association with an inferior infarct. Surgery is indicated for cases causing severe heart failure unresponsive to drug treatment.
- *Ventricular septal defect*. This occurs after about 1% of infarcts, and is more common with anteroseptal than inferior infarction. It is due to rupture of a softened area of the septum, and is signalled by the development of a new systolic murmur at the lower left sternal edge, usually with cardiac failure that is often fatal. Surgical repair may be attempted, but there is a dilemma about the timing of operation. Although it is generally contended that the best results are obtained with surgery about 2 weeks after the infarct, by which time some healing has occurred, in fact some possibly salvable patients die whilst waiting for operation.
- *The post-cardiac injury syndrome (also known as Dressler's syndrome)*. This is discussed on page 146.
- *Cardiac aneurysm*. This is ballooning during systole of an area of damaged heart muscle. It is usually symptomless but may predispose to cardiac failure, arterial embolus or recurrent ventricular arrhythmias. It is suggested by paradoxical lateral displacement of the cardiac apex during systole and persistence of ST elevation on ECG, and may be demonstrated by:
  a chest x-ray and cardiac screening,
  b isotope gated scanning of the heart (see page 40), or
  c left ventricular angiogram (see page 41).

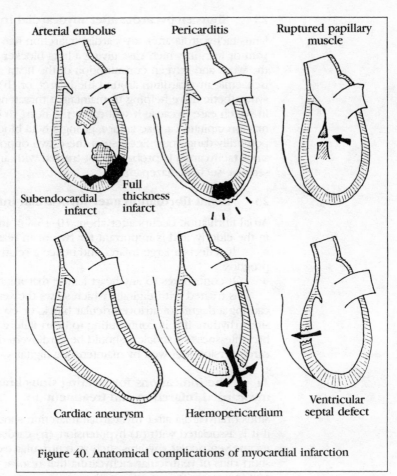

Figure 40. Anatomical complications of myocardial infarction

● *Haemopericardium*. This occurs in about 2% of patients, and is due to rupture of a softened area of infarction. It causes acute cardiac tamponade and is usually fatal.

● *Angina afterwards*. This occurs in about 20% of patients. Its management is discussed on pages 103 and 132.

21 Ventricular extrasystoles after myocardial infarction

It used to be thought that ventricular extrasystoles or premature beats in the hours or days after an infarct indicated increased excitability of the heart muscle indicative of impending ventricular fibrillation—hence the term 'warning arrhythmia'. However, it is now appreciated that ventricular fibrillation occurs as often in patients with uninterrupted sinus rhythm as in those with ectopic activity, and that such activity is probably not of any great prognostic significance although some authorities regard ventricular ectopics occurring on the preceding T wave (R on T) as a warning arrhythmia.

22   Sinus tachycardia after myocardial infarction

Sinus tachycardia after myocardial infarction may be due to (a) pain or fear, in which case giving a beta blocker drug may reduce the work and oxygen consumption of the heart and help preserve ischaemic myocardium around the infarct, or (b) to compensatory sympathetic drive helping to maintain a threatened cardiac output, in which case because it will cause the heart to beat less hard and may precipitate cardiac failure, giving a beta blocking drug is potentilly dangerous. Because of these two opposites, on balance sinus tachycardia is probably best treated with an opiate or sedative such as diazepam.

23   Atrial fibrillation after myocardial infarction

Atrial fibrillation occurs after about 10–15% of infarcts, especially in the elderly, and is important for two main reasons:
●   It reflects a large infarct and hence a relatively poor prognosis.
●   It contributes to any heart failure that might be present.
    It is treated with digitalis which slows the ventricular rate by causing a degree of atrioventricular block, or even converts it to sinus rhythm. If it is contributing to heart failure with associated breathlessness or shock it should be cardioverted with DC cardioversion followed by maintenance digitalis.

24   The indications for treating sinus bradycardia after myocardial infarction and treatment

Sinus bradycardia after myocardial infarction should be treated only if it is associated with (a) hypotension, (b) cardiac failure, or (c) escape ventricular rhythms such as ventricular extrasystoles or short runs of ventricular tachycardia that resolve when the heart rate increases. Treatment is with atropine given intravenously in a dose of 0.3 mg which may be repeated as necessary after 15 minutes. As discussed below, very occasionally pacing may be necessary.

25   The indications for a temporary pacemaker after myocardial infarction

●   *Anterior infarction complicated by complete heart block*
The reason for this is that, as discussed on page 110, to cause complete heart block an anterior infarct must be very large, extending from the front of the heart back into the septum to involve the conducting tissue. An infarct of such a size is a threat to stroke volume. An adequate heart rate is therefore required to ensure an adequate cardiac output, and in the presence of complete heart block can be achieved only by pacing.
●   *An unwell patient with an inferior infarct complicated by complete heart block.* As implied on page 110, complete heart block is commoner but less of a threat with inferior infarction. In this situation, it is therefore reasonable to observe a patient who is

well, although pacing should be carried out if there is evidence of heart failure such as hypotension or breathlessness, or if the pulse rate is much less than 50 beats per minute.

With inferior infarction *lesser forms of heart block* of the first and second degree types and bundle branch block can usually be safely observed. However, the situation is *potentially* different in cases in which these lesser forms of heart block and bundle branch block occur with anterior infarction. The reason for this is that these lesser forms of heart block and bundle branch block may be harbingers of complete heart block which, as discussed above, in the presence of an anterior infarct implies a large infarct that would be a threat to life if complete heart block were to occur. For this reason some authorities recommend *prophylactic* insertion of a pacing wire for anterior infarction complicated by first or second degree heart block or sinus rhythm with left anterior hemi-block and right bundle branch block (see page 61).

● Occasionally it may be necessary to pace a patient with symptomatic sinus bradycardia that is unresponsive to atropine and causing hypotension or cardiac failure.

Shock: definition and causes; the shocked patient; cardiogenic shock following myocardial infarction

Question

26i Define the term shock.

ii List the various causes of shock. Describe the underlying mechanisms in anaphylactic shock and septicaemic shock. List the main vasoactive substances involved in their generation.

iii Describe the clinical picture of a shocked patient.

iv What is the mortality of cardiogenic shock after myocardial infarction? How might you attempt to treat it?

Answer

26 Shock

i *Definition.* Shock is a syndrome characterised by circulatory insufficiency resulting in inadequate perfusion of the tissues which if prolonged leads to cellular dysfunction.

ii *Causes of shock.*

● *Failure of the pumping action of the heart* due for instance to myocardial infarction, or an arrhythmia such as very fast atrial fibrillation, atrial flutter, ventricular tachycardia or ventricular fibrillation.

● *Blood or fluid loss* due for instance to haemorrhage, dehydration or a burn.

● *Obstruction of the circulation* due for instance to a pulmonary embolus obstructing the pulmonary artery, cardiac tamponade or tension pneumothorax.

● *Deranged vascular tone* due for instance to a simple faint, anaphylaxis or septicaemia. In a simple faint the underlying mechanism is vagotonia causing bradycardia and loss of sympathetic tone causing pooling of blood in venous capacitance vessels in the limbs and gut.

In anaphylactic and septicaemic shock the main mechanisms are (a) loss of vascular smooth muscle tone leading to vasodilatation, and (b) an increase of capillary permeability leading to loss of protein and fluid from the vascular compartment.

In anaphylactic shock this occurs mainly as a result of activation of mast cells and release of vasoactive substances such as histamine, prostaglandins, leukotrienes and bradykinin—all of which affect vascular tone and permeability.

In septicaemic shock a similar effect is brought about by bacterial toxins causing direct damage to cell walls and activation of the following systems:

● Complement with production of the vasoactive substances, factors C3a and C5a.

● Mast and other cells with production of the vasoactive substances histamine, prostaglandins, leukotrienes and bradykinin.

● ACTH/endorphin from the anterior pituitary gland with production of ß-endorphin that probably has similar effects on the vasculature to morphine, causing pooling of blood in venous capacitance vessels in the limbs and gut, and hypotension.

● In addition, in some cases of septicaemic shock the microcirculation is obstructed by amorphous masses of fibrin, platelets and blood cells as a result of activation of the coagulation/fibrinolytic system causing intravascular coagulation.

iii   *Clinically* a patient suffering from shock of any cause appears ill, and sometimes confused, restless or apathetic. There may be air hunger. Usually the periphery is cold and cyanosed due to poor perfusion, and the pulse weak and blood pressure low, but in some cases of septicaemic shock the cardiac output is normal or even high and the periphery warm although perfusion of the tissues is poor. This is due to shunting of blood through precapillary arteriovenous anastomoses.

iv   *Cardiogenic shock following myocardial infarction* has a mortality of 85–90%. The aim of treatment of all forms of shock is to restore tissue perfusion. In the case of cardiogenic shock following myocardial infarction this is by attempting to increase cardiac output. Traditionally positive inotropic drugs such as dopamine, dobutamine or salbutamol are given, but probably do not improve the prognosis. Balloon counter pulsation, in which a balloon is placed in the aorta and inflated in diastole causing increased blood to flow to the coronary arteries (which normally receive blood in diastole), may sustain a shocked patient with a surgically correctable complication such as an incompetent mitral valve, cardiac aneurysm or ventricular septal defect, until surgery can be undertaken. Each inflation of the balloon increases the cardiac output by about 30 ml.

Rehabilitation and long-term treatment

Questions

27   Discuss the main features of the rehabilitation of patients who have suffered a myocardial infarction.
28   What is the role of beta blocking drugs and of aspirin in the first year or so after myocardial infarction?
29   What is the rationale of exercise testing after myocardial infarction?

Answers

27   Rehabilitation

Because a heart attack is a frightening experience that is perceived by most people as a threat to life after the event is over, patients need active encouragement to return to as full a life as possible. For convenience this is most easily considered by dividing the subject into personal aspects and medical aspects.

● *Personal aspects*. For those who have made a complete physical recovery the aim is a return to full activity over the 6–8 weeks following the onset of the illness. For about 2 weeks the patient should dress each day but spend much of the time resting; thereafter activity may gradually increase. Driving may be resumed after 4 weeks, and work, perhaps initally part-time, after 8 weeks. The need for adequate relaxation and rest should be emphasised. Some centres run rehabilitation exercise programmes. Although it is unlikely that these affect the prognosis they do improve patients' confidence and sense of well being. Because many patients are apprehensive about the vigorous activity it involves, counselling about sexual activity should be given with a view to a return to the patient's previous pattern of behaviour. Often a word of reassurance is all that is needed.

For those who are left with cardiac failure or angina these guidelines need to be modified according to the degree of disability.

● *Medical aspects*. Because the risk of sudden death is halved in those who stop smoking, all smokers should be persuaded to stop smoking. The blood pressure should be checked and if found, hypertension should be treated. Unless they are elderly, the prognosis and need for further investigation of those who appear to have made a complete recovery should be assessed by an exercise test. The rationale behind this is discussed in the answer to question 29. Prophylaxis with a beta blocking drug and aspirin should be prescribed as discussed in the answer to the next question. Because they are temporarily deranged by an illness such as myocardial infarction, plasma lipids should be measured after a period of about 3 months, and any dietary or other measures taken as necessary.

Patients left with cardiac failure should be investigated for surgically remediable causes such as cardiac aneurysm or valvular disease, and treated along the lines suggested on page 43. As suggested in the answer to question 29, patients left with angina are at particular risk and in most cases should undergo coronary arteriography with a view to possible coronary artery bypass surgery.

28 Beta blocking drugs and aspirin after myocardial infarction

Several trials have demonstrated that in patients aged less than 70 who have suffered an uncomplicated myocardial infarct, daily administration of a beta blocking drug reduces mortality in the first year or so after the illness by about 20%, that is from about 10% to 8%, saving about two lives for every 100 patients treated. Much of this benefit is due to a reduction in sudden death suggesting that the drugs act as an anti-arrhythmic. Because of this a beta blocking drug such as timolol, sotalol, atenolol or propranolol should be given for a year or two to all patients aged less than 70 who have sustained a myocardial infarct, provided beta blockers are not contraindicated for reasons such as bronchial asthma, incipient cardiac failure, bradycardia or low blood pressure.

Similarly, prophylaxis with a regular small dose of aspirin has been shown to reduce the long-term mortality of myocardial infarction by about one for every 100 patients treated, and also to prevent a recurrence of non-fatal infarction in another. How many years aspirin should be taken for, and whether beta blocking drugs and aspirin have an added prophylactic effect is not known.

29 Exercise testing after myocardial infarction

Apart from patients who are left with heart failure and are therefore at an increased risk, it has been shown that after myocardial infarction patients who appear to have made a complete recovery may be grouped by their response to an exercise test into those with a poor prognosis who develop anginal-like chest pain or ECG evidence of reversible ischaemia whilst exercising, and those with a good prognosis who are able to exercise without chest pain or ECG changes. Studies are proceeding to identify whether interventions such as coronary artery bypass improve the prognosis of those shown by the exercise test to have a poor outlook. Whilst the results are awaited, currently many such patients are being referred for coronary arteriography and possible coronary artery bypass surgery.

Further Reading

AIMS Trial Study Group (1988). Effect of intravenous APSAC on mortality after acute myocardial infarction: preliminary report of a placebo controlled clinical trial. *Lancet i*, 545–9.

Braunwald E (ed) (1984). *Heart Disease*, 2nd edition. WB Saunders, Philadelphia. Chapters 36, pathological and clinical manifestations; 37, management of acute myocardial infarction.

Gruppo Italiano per lo Studio Della Streptochinasi Nell' Infarcto
    Miocardico (GISSI) (1987). Longterm effects of intravenous
    thrombolysis in acute myocardial infarction: final report of
    the Gissi Study. *Lancet ii*, 871-4.
Hampton JR (1986). *The ECG Made Easy*, 3rd edition. Churchill
    Livingstone, Edinburgh.
ISIS-1 (First International Study of Infarct Survival) collaborative
    group (1986). Randomized trial of intravenous atenolol
    among 16,027 cases of suspected acute myocardial infarction.
    Lancet ii, 57-65.
ISIS-2 (Second International Study of Infarct Survival) collaborative
    group (1988). Randomized trial of intravenous streptokinase,
    oral aspirin, both, or neither among 17,187 cases of
    suspected acute myocardial infarction. *Lancet ii*, 349-60.
Norwegian Multicenter Study Group (1981). Timolol-induced
    reduction in mortality and reinfarction in patients surviving
    acute myocardial infarction. *N.Engl.J.Med. 304*, 801-7.
Shaper AG, Pocock SJ (1987). Risk factors for ischaemic heart
    disease in British men. *Br. Heart J.* 57, 11-16.

Case E

A Case of Chest Pain — No. 3: Mr A-M, aged 43 years

A happily married man who smoked 70 cigarettes per day and worked under great pressure as the sales manager of an engineering firm that was expanding its export trade. His wife was 7 months pregnant with their third child.

History of present condition

Whilst recovering in an ordinary ward, 3 days after transfer from the coronary care unit where he had been admitted with a full thickness inferolateral myocardial infarct, Mr A-M suddenly woke at 5 a.m., complained of further central chest pain and slumped back unconscious on the bed, having suffered a cardiac arrest.

Chapter 7
Cardiac Arrest in Hospital

The arrest team; differential diagnosis

Questions

1   How many people should be in the cardiac arrest team? Who should they be? Who should be in charge of the team? What should be the duties of each member of the team?
2   What arrhythmias are likely to cause a cardiac arrest?
3   What other causes of unconsciousness are sometimes confused with cardiac arrest?

Answers

1   The cardiac arrest team

Every doctor, nurse and member of staff who works in a clinical area should be proficient at cardiac resuscitation. In hospital the resuscitation team should consist of at least two, and preferably three doctors, of whom one should be an anaesthetist and another a physician. Other members of the team should include a senior nurse from the coronary care or intensive care unit or an operating department assistant (ODA), one other senior nurse and a hospital porter to bring the emergency trolley. Each member of the team should know exactly what is required of them. Details of the arrest procedure are given below, but in general the anaesthetist, senior nurse or ODA should attend to the airway and intubation if that proves necessary, whilst the other nurse attends to the cardiac massage. The physician should attend to the defibrillator and recording the heart rhythm.

One of the doctors must be very clearly in charge. Although he or she should help with the resuscitation they should tend to stand back and have an overall view of what is happening. The time that the resuscitation call is given out should be noted as it is happening. Once at the site of the arrest a nurse or other member of the ward staff should be instructed to keep a written timed record of events and treatments. All idle onlookers should be sent away.

2   The arrhythmias likely to cause cardiac arrest

These are ventricular fibrillation or tachycardia and asystole. Occasionally the rhythm may be sinus rhythm without any perceptible cardiac output—a terminal condition known as electromechanical dissociation.

3   Other causes of unconsciousness that are sometimes confused with cardiac arrest

The specific sign of cardiac arrest is pulselessness. If the pulse is present the cause of the unconsciousness is some other condition such as a faint, hypoglycaemic attack or epileptic seizure. If the pulse is present but the patient is not breathing the cause of unconsciousness is respiratory arrest due to conditions such as asthma, carbon dioxide narcosis in a blue bloating chronic bronchitic, or the effects of too large a dose of a sedative.

Assessment and management
Questions

4   How is cardiac arrest confirmed? Assuming the diagnosis is confirmed what should be done immediately, even before cardiac massage is initiated?
5   What is the alphabet, the A, B, C, D, E, of cardiac arrest not responding to the steps mentioned in the answer to question 4? Explain the action that is implied by each of the above letters of the alphabet.

Answers

4   Confirmation of cardiac arrest, and the steps that should be taken at once

The diagnosis is established by two signs: unconsciousness, and absence of the carotid or femoral pulse. As soon as the diagnosis is confirmed, before proceeding to cardiac massage, a single blow should be given to the precordium from a height of about 15-20 cm with the side of the clenched fist. Sometimes this will convert ventricular fibrillation, ventricular tachycardia or asystole to sinus rhythm, and should be tried in all cases. If the pulse is not immediately restored and if the patient does not immediately show signs of regaining consciousness life support must be provided along the lines indicated by the letters A, B, C below. Until the arrival of the arrest team this will be by the ward nurses or whichever members of the staff happen to be present.

The only exception is that if a defibrillator is *immediately* available and if the arrest has occurred in the coronary care or intensive care unit or other area where trained staff are available, the rhythm of the heart should be quickly ascertained and ventricular fibrillation or tachycardia cardioverted without wasting time giving cardiac massage.

5   The A, B, C, D, E of cardiac arrest not responding to the steps mentioned above

If a thump on the chest is ineffective and the defibrillator is not immediately to hand full cardiac resuscitation is necessary and is most easily organised according to the letters A, B, C, D, E.
●   *A = assess.* As has already been mentioned, the cardinal

signs of cardiac arrest are unconsciousness and absence of the carotid or femoral pulse. Unconsciousness should be checked by shouting at the patient 'Are you alright?' and by gentle shaking.

An airway should be established by tilting the patient's head backwards, fully extending the neck and removing any vomitus or foreign material from the pharynx. Extending the neck this way lifts the tongue off the posterior wall of the pharynx.

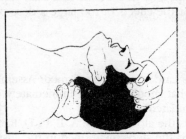 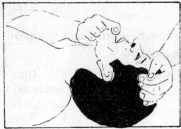

Figure 41.
Establishing an airway

● *B = breathing*. Three methods of emergency ventilation are available:

a *Mouth to mouth ventilation*. This is given by taking a deep breath, pinching the patient's nose, and blowing forcefully into the mouth.

b *Brook airway*. This is a simple device consisting of a tube with a one way valve, a flange to fit over the patient's lips and a tongue depressor. By separating the patient and the attendant blowing into the lungs it facilitates ventilation in a more aesthetic way than mouth to mouth resuscitation.

c *Bag valve mask*. The advantage of this is that it allows the delivery of oxygen, and also allows the operator to stand back.

In each instance an airtight seal must be ensured and the chest seen to rise and fall, otherwise ventilation is inadequate.

If the initial attempt to restore the heart beat is unsuccessful an *endotracheal tube* should be inserted. Proficiency at intubation should be gained by practising with a resuscitation manikin or by attending anaesthetic sessions.

● *C = circulation*. External cardiac massage is given by placing the heel of one hand over the lower half of the sternum and covering it with the other hand. Keeping the arms straight the sternum is then compressed at a rate of eighty compressions per minute. Each compression should be of the same length of time as each relaxation. The changes of intrathoracic pressure thus created alternately squeeze and relax the heart, simulating a heart beat and propelling blood into the arteries where the result should be checked by palpating the carotid or femoral pulse. If there are two operators the massage should be interrupted every five cycles so that the lungs may be ventilated once. When only one operator is

present the massage should be interrupted every 10 cycles and the lungs ventilated twice.
- *D = drip*. If the resuscitation continues for more than a minute or two an intravenous dextrose/saline drip should be set up. Speed is of the essence. If an arm vein is not immediately accessible, the subclavian or internal jugular vein should be cannulated.
- *E = ECG*. The paddles of a modern defibrillator may be used as ECG leads to ascertain quickly the rhythm of the heart, and when indicated should be used to cardiovert the patient as quickly as possible.

Specific aspects of management
Questions

6   How is ventricular fibrillation or life threatening ventricular tachycardia treated? To what level should the defibrillator be charged? How is ventricular fibrillation resistant to the standard charge treated? What would you do if you were uncertain if the rhythm was fine ventricular fibrillation or asystole?
7   How is asystole treated? What drugs are used in its treatment?
8   What is the concentration of sodium bicarbonate used for cardiac resuscitation? What is special about this concentration? How much sodium bicarbonate is usually given during a cardiac arrest?
9   What specific treatment should be given after a successful resuscitation?

Answers

6   **The treatment of ventricular fibrillation or life threatening ventricular tachycardia**

This is by immediate defibrillation with a charge of 200 joules. Although ventricular tachycardia may respond to anti-arrhythmic medication, ventricular fibrillation does not. The only effective treatment of ventricular fibrillation is therefore electrical defibrillation causing depolarisation of all the myocardial cells that are not in the refractory period. This breaks the fibrillatory waveforms and allows the normal impulse to take over control of the heart beat.

If 200 joules fails to restore a satisfactory rhythm defibrillation should be repeated with a charge of 400 joules. If still unsuccessful lignocaine 100 mg should be given intravenously or via the endotracheal tube and any acidosis corrected as described below. If the arrhythmia still persists an alternative anti-arrhythmic such as disopyramide or mexiletine may be tried. In cases that are still persistent, defibrillation may be successful after the administration of 5-10 ml of 1 in 10 000 adrenaline either intravenously or via the endotracheal tube.

If there is doubt about whether the rhythm is fine ventricular fibrillation or asystole, it should be assumed to be ventricular fibrillation and the patient defibrillated.

7   The treatment of asystole

If external cardiac massage does not quickly restore a heart rhythm, 10 ml of 10% calcium gluconate or calcium chloride should be given intravenously together with 10 ml of 1 in 10 000 adrenaline either intravenously or via the endotracheal tube, and any acidosis corrected as described below.

8   Sodium bicarbonate

The most important way of reversing acidosis is by adequate ventilation. However, a small quantity of sodium bicarbonate should be given. The concentration used for cardiac arrest is 8.4%. The special feature of this concentration is that 1 ml = 1 mmol. The volume administered is usually 50 ml, i.e. 50 mmol.

9   Treatment after successful resuscitation

This will depend upon the rhythm causing the arrest and the condition of the patient after the resuscitation.

After ventricular fibrillation or tachycardia lignocaine or another class I anti-arrhythmic should be given. After asystole, unless due to anoxia or some other readily reversible cause, a prophylactic temporary pacemaker should be inserted. If the level of consciousness is impaired intravenous dexamethasone 4 mg 6 hourly for three to four doses, and frusemide 40–80 mg should be given to minimise cerebral oedema. If respiration is insufficient, the patient should be ventilated mechanically.

Further Reading

Braunwald E (ed) (1984). *Heart Disease*, 2nd edition. WB Saunders, Philadelphia. Chapter 22, cardiovascular collapse and sudden cardiac death.

Case F   # A Case of Chest Pain — No. 4: Mr H-V, aged 29 years

A happily married builder's labourer living in his own small modern terraced house with his wife and two young children.

History of present condition

Visited urgently at home at the request of his general practitioner with a history of being well until a week previously, when he developed a typical 'flu-like' illness with a high temperature, feelings of being unwell and aching of his muscles.

Initially he improved, but after 3 days he became unwell again with increasing breathlessness and severe pains over the left lower anterior chest. The pain was continuous, but worse with coughing and with lying flat at night. It was eased by sitting up and leaning forward.

Past medical history

Nil of note.

Family history

Nil of note.

Relevant direct questions

Sputum: nil.
Swelling of ankles: nil.
Smoking: 20 cigarettes per day.
Drugs: His general practitioner had prescribed dihydrocodeine for his chest pain, and had also prescribed courses of the antibiotics ampicillin and co-trimoxazole.

Mr H-V

Questions

1   Pain of this type is said to be pleuritic. What are the main differential diagnoses of pleuritic chest pain?
2   What condition does the history suggest Mr H-V was suffering from?
3   What clinical signs might you have expected to find on examining him?

Answers

1   The main differential diagnoses of pleuritic chest pain

● *Pain from the musculoskeletal system* due to conditions such as torn muscle fibres, cracked or fractured ribs, Bornholm disease and the other conditions listed on page 85.

● *Pain from the pleura due to:*

a   *Primary conditions of the pleura* such as viral pleurisy caused by Coxsackie B virus and pleural tumours such as mesothelioma.

b   *Secondary conditions of the pleura* in which pleural involvement is due to respiratory or circulatory problems such as pneumonia, carcinoma of the bronchus, pulmonary infarction and the post-cardiac injury syndrome.

● *Pain due to inflammation of the pericardium*, i.e. pericarditis.

● *Pain due to inflammation and movement of the peritoneum with respiration*. This will usually be felt in the upper abdomen or lower chest, and for example may be due to:

a   *Peritonitis* resulting from inflammation or rupture of an intra-abdominal organ.

b   *Hepatic metastases* invading or stretching the peritoneum covering the liver.

2   The condition from which Mr H-V was suffering

The history of pleuritic chest pain at the front of the lower chest, made worse by lying down, and eased by sitting up and leaning forward is pathognomonic of *acute pericarditis.*

3   The clinical signs that Mr H-V might have been expected to show

● *A pericardial rub*. This is the main physical sign of acute pericarditis, and is typically a scratching sound like the rubbing of sandpaper and may consist of presystole, systolic and diastolic components. It is best heard to the left of the lower sternum. Because of its high pitched quality it often sounds 'nearer' to the listener than a murmur.

● *Signs at the base of the left lung*. In some cases of acute pericarditis there may also be an associated pneumonitis and effusion at the base of the left lung—a condition known as Ewart's sign.

● *If cardiac tamponade* is present there may be signs associated with this. Details of these are given on page 146.

In MR H-V's case physical examination revealed a pale, tall, muscular, unwell-looking young man, temperature 38.5°C. There was a loud pericardial rub. Otherwise clinical examination was normal except for arterial pulsus paradoxus, 8 mmHg, BP 130/80 lying and standing.

Chapter 8
Pericardial Disease

Aetiology
Questions

1   What are the three main clinical conditions or diseases of the pericardium?
2   List the main causes of pericardial disease.

Answers

1   The three main clinical conditions of the pericardium

- Acute pericarditis
- Pericardial tamponade
- Chronic constrictive pericarditis

2   The main causes of pericardial disease

- *Infective*
a   *Viral.* The specific viruses are listed on page 145. When a virus is suspected, but not proven by isolation or serology, and when no other cause is evident, the condition is often referred to as *acute idiopathic pericarditis.*
b   *Bacterial.* Usually secondary to cardiac surgery, immunosuppression, rupture of the oesophagus, or pneumococcal pneumonia.
c   *Tuberculosis.* This may present as acute pericarditis, although more commonly it presents as a chronic condition. There may be no other evidence of tuberculosis, but in some cases symptoms of a systemic illness such as fever, anorexia, lethargy and weight loss may be present.
- *Myocardial infarction.* Either during the acute phase of the illness due to involvement of the pericardium in the infarct or as part of the post-cardiac injury syndrome.
- *Post-cardiac injury syndrome.* Details of this are given on page 146.
- *Rheumatic fever.* In this situation pericarditis is usually associated with evidence of rheumatic carditis.
- *Uraemia.* Even occasionally in patients receiving haemodialysis.
- *Collagenoses*, for example:
Systemic lupus erythematosus (SLE)
Rheumatoid arthritis (RA)
Scleroderma
Polyarteritis nodosa (PAN)

• *Drugs causing an SLE-like syndrome*, for example:
Hydrallazine
Procainamide
Isoniazid
Minoxidil
• *Neoplasia* due to
a   *Invasion* from an adjacent primary carcinoma of the
bronchus, or from secondary deposits due to leukaemia, or
tumours such as carcinoma of the breast or lymphoma.
b   *Irradiation*. As a side effect of irradiating tumours within
the thorax, especially tumours within the mediastinum.
• *Haemorrhage within the pericardium* due to:
Anticoagulants
Following cardiac surgery
Dissection of an aortic aneurysm
• *Hypothyroidism*. Rare and usually asymptomatic, invariably
resolving with treatment of the hypothyroidism.

Acute pericarditis
Questions

3   List the triad of symptoms, signs and investigations used in
the recognition of a typical case of acute pericarditis.
4   What are the characteristics of the typical pain of
pericarditis?
5   Describe the characteristics of a pericardial rub.
6   Describe the typical ECG changes found in (i) acute
pericarditis, (ii) pericardial effusion.
7   Which viruses may cause acute pericarditis? Which age
groups are patients affected by viral pericarditis likely to come
from? What is the likelihood of it recurring? How may it be
treated?
8i   List the clinical features of the post-cardiac injury syndrome.
  ii   List the conditions causing it.
  iii   Describe its pathophysiology, i.e. the mechanism by which it
is thought to be caused.
  iv   How may it be treated?

Answers

3   **The triad used in the recognition of a typical case of
acute pericarditis**

• The characteristic pain
• The pericardial rub
• The characteristic ECG changes

4   **The characteristics of the typical pain of acute
pericarditis**

These were discussed on page 142, and are pleuritic chest pain at
the front of the lower chest, made worse by lying flat, and eased
by sitting up and leaning forward or adopting some other
particular position.

5 The characteristics of a pericardial rub

These were also discussed on page 142, and are a scratching sound like the rubbing of sandpaper, which may have presystolic, systolic and diastolic components. It is best heard to the left of the lower sternum. Because of its high pitched quality it often sounds 'nearer' to the listener than a murmur.

6 The typical ECG changes associated with acute pericarditis and pericardial effusion

i   *Acute pericarditis:*
●   Concave ST elevation, like the back of a saddle occurs in most leads except aVr.
●   After a few days the ST elevation resolves, to be replaced by inversion of the T wave.
●   Sometimes the above changes are accompanied by atrial premature beats or atrial fibrillation.

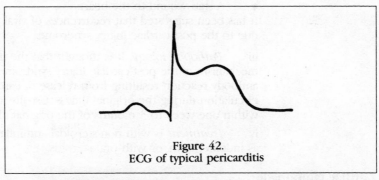

Figure 42.
ECG of typical pericarditis

ii   *Pericardial effusion:*
●   Sinus tachycardia is the commonest finding, often in association with low voltage QRS complexes that are a result of the fluid within the pericardium inhibiting the conduction of impulses to the recording electrodes.
●   Occasionally electrical alternans may occur, and consists of alternating complexes of differing morphology due to the heart swinging freely within the pericardial fluid.

7 Viral pericarditis

●   This may be caused by any of the following viruses:
Coxsackie A or B
Influenza
Echo 8
Herpes simplex
Chickenpox
Adenovirus
●   Persons of all ages may be affected, especially young adults.
●   It may recur for up to 2 years in as many as a quarter of cases.
●   Usually the erythrocyte sedimentation rate (ESR) is elevated,

and there is often a neutrophilia followed by a lymphophilia.
● Treatment is with non-steroidal anti-inflammatory drugs (NSAID), such as indomethacin, or with oral steroids such as prednisolone.

8 The post-cardiac injury syndrome

i Clinically this is characterised by:
● Pyrexia
● Pericarditis } the three 'P's
● Pleurisy

● Elevated ESR
Arthralgia may also develop.

ii It may follow:
● Myocardial infarction when it is known as Dressler's syndrome.
● Cardiac surgery
● A stab wound to the heart.
It has been suggested that recurrences of viral pericarditis may be due to the post-cardiac injury syndrome.

iii *Pathophysiology*. It is thought that the underlying mechanism of the post-cardiac injury syndrome is an antigen/ antibody reaction resulting from release of cardiac antigen into the circulation during the original illness. Usually it manifests itself within one week to 3 months of the original illness.

iv *Treatment* is with non-steroidal anti-inflammatory drugs such as indomethacin, or with oral steroids.

Cardiac tamponade
Questions

9 What is cardiac tamponade?
10 Describe its pathophysiology, i.e. the two mechanisms by which it produces the symptoms and signs with which it is associated.
11 What are the symptoms and signs of cardiac tamponade?
12 What is arterial pulsus paradoxus? How is it measured, and by what mechanisms is it thought to be caused? With what conditions other than cardiac tamponade may it be associated?
13 What is venous paradoxus or Kussmaul's sign? By what mechanism is it thought to be caused?
14 How is cardiac tamponade investigated?
15 How may it be treated?

Answers

9 Definition

Cardiac tamponade is a clinical condition resulting from the effects of fluid within the pericardial space interfering with filling of the ventricles during diastole.

10 The pathophysiology or mechanisms by which cardiac tamponade produces the symptoms and signs with which it is associated

The tightly contained layer of fluid around the heart interferes with filling of the ventricles during diastole causing:
- *Low cardiac output* with a small stroke volume, compensatory tachycardia, and a reduced output of urine.
- *Restricted venous return* resulting in venous congestion.

11 Symptoms and signs

These follow from the low cardiac output and from the venous congestion.

Due to the reduced cardiac output, the main *symptom* is breathlessness.

The main *signs* are:
- *A small volume pulse* with sinus tachycardia. In about half the cases the systolic blood pressure is < 100 mmHg.
- *In the neck the jugular venous pulse* is markedly raised with exaggeration of the x descent. A full description of the various waves and descents in the JVP is given on page 15. Sometimes venous paradoxus or Kussmaul's sign is also present, and is described below.
- *The apex beat is usually impalpable*. If palpable, typically it is inside the lateral border of cardiac dullness.
- *The heart sounds are quiet*. As a result of the low cardiac output the heart valves close with a low velocity that as explained on page 18 generates very little sound. In addition, any fluid in front of the heart interferes with the conduction of sound to the stethoscope.
- *Arterial pulsus paradoxus*. This is described below.

12 Arterial pulsus paradoxus

This is an exaggeration of the normal variation of systolic blood pressure during the respiratory cycle and is not in any way paradoxical. With significant pulsus paradoxus the systolic blood pressure falls 10 mmHg or more during inspiration. It may be found in about half the cases of cardiac tamponade, and occasionally may be so marked as to be obvious during palpation of the radial pulse. However, in the majority of cases it is most easily determined by using a sphygmomanometer to record the variation of systolic blood pressure throughout the respiratory cycle.

The cause of pulsus paradoxus is not fully understood, although at least two mechanisms have been proposed. Common to each is the fact that the tightly contained fluid within the pericardial sac obstructs venous return to the heart and cardiac filling.
- According to the first mechanism, as inspiration proceeds and the lungs expand, the pressure within the thorax and its contents falls in the normal way. The fall of pressure this causes in

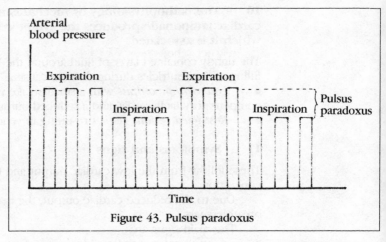

Figure 43. Pulsus paradoxus

the pulmonary veins may result in the pressure within these veins falling to levels that are less than the abnormal pressure within the heart as it sits in the tightly contained pericardial sac. As a consequence, during inspiration the flow of blood from the pulmonary veins to the heart is reduced or even reversed, causing a temporary reduction of cardiac output and blood pressure. During expiration the increased pressure that occurs in the thorax and pulmonary veins is sufficient to drive blood forward into the heart, restoring cardiac output and blood pressure.

● During expiration the diaphragm is at its highest and the fluid filled pericardial sac almost spherical. As the diaphragm descends during inspiration the pericardial sac elongates and its volume decreases. This results in a further increase of pressure within the sac that further obstructs the flow of blood into the right atrium from the great veins, and into the left atrium from the pulmonary veins, augmenting what has been said in the paragraph above. As a consequence venous return to both sides of the heart is further decreased, adding to the fall of cardiac output during inspiration. Obstruction of this type on the right side of the heart probably accounts for Kussmaul's sign, described below.

Other causes of arterial pulsus paradoxus

● Airways obstruction   { Asthma
                           Chronic obstructive airways
                           disease (COAD)

● Hypovolaemic shock
● Cardiac failure

13   Venous paradoxus or Kussmaul's sign

This is a paradoxical increase of jugular venous distension during inspiration causing the neck to become visibly enlarged. Normally, of course, any jugular venous distension decreases during inspiration as blood is drawn into the thorax. In those cases in which venous paradoxus occurs the descent of the diaphragm during inspiration causes the pressure within the fluid filled pericardial sac, and hence the right atrium, to increase to levels that obstruct venous return from the great veins.

14 Investigation of cardiac tamponade

● *ECG.* The changes were described on page 145 and consist of sinus tachycardia, often with low voltage QRS complexes, and sometimes electrical alternans.

● *Chest x-ray.* Typically this shows a large globular shaped heart that may be indistinguishable from the heart of a cardiomyopathy. However, with pericardial effusion the lung fields are characteristically *clear*, whereas with left ventricular failure due to cardiomyopathy the lung fields are typically *congested*.

● *Echocardiography.* This shows an echo free space occupied by fluid between the visceral and parietal layers of the pericardium behind the heart. With large effusions a similar space may be seen in front of the heart.

● *Cardiac catheterisation.* Usually this is not necessary. If performed it reveals that the end diastolic pressure within each of the four chambers of the heart is the same to within 5 mmHg. In addition an increase in the distance between the outside of the cardiac silhouette and the outline of the left or right ventricular cavities may be demonstrated by the injection of contrast medium.

15 Treatment of cardiac tamponade

This comprises two main aspects:

● *Resuscitation.* If the tamponade is embarrassing the patient and causing severe arterial hypotension it may be necessary first to resuscitate the patient by giving an infusion of normal saline in an attempt to increase cardiac output.

● *Pericardiocentesis* (needle aspiration) is then performed, using either the apical or xiphisternal approaches. If the needle is connected to an ECG lead ST elevation on the cardiograph will indicate that the needle has touched the myocardium in which case it should be withdrawn a little.

Blood stained pericardial fluid can be differentiated from blood from the left ventricle by (a) its dark colour, and (b) its failure to clot.

Chronic constrictive pericarditis

Questions

16 What is chronic constrictive pericarditis?

17 Describe its pathophysiology, i.e. the two mechanisms by which it produces the symptoms and signs with which it is associated.

18 List the ways in which the typical symptoms and signs of chronic constrictive pericarditis differ from those of cardiac tamponade.

19   What effects may chronic constrictive pericarditis have on other organs?
20   How is chronic constrictive pericarditis investigated?
21   How may it be treated?
22   List the differential diagnosis of ascites?

Answers

16   Definition

Chronic constrtictive pericarditis is a clinical condition due to scarring and contraction of the pericardium around the heart interfering with filling of the ventricles during diastole.

17   Pathophysiology

The mechanisms by which chronic constrictive pericarditis produces the symptoms and signs with which it is associated follow from the interference of ventricular filling during diastole, and are:
● *Low cardiac output*.
● *Restricted venous return* causing venous congestion, in this case augmented by chronic sodium retention.

18   The main differences in the symptoms and signs of chronic constrictive pericarditis and cardiac tamponade

The typical symptoms and signs of cardiac tamponade are described on page 146. By way of contrast, in chronic constrictive pericarditis the following are the characteristic findings.
● *Ascites* rather than breathlessness, although there may be some orthopnoea and breathlessness on exertion. The ascites is due mainly to a combination of increased venous pressure and sodium retention.
● However, despite the ascites, *oedema of the legs is not marked*.
● *Marked wasting of the muscles of the limbs* is often present, and combined with the ascites may mistakenly suggest malignancy.
● *Slight arterial pulsus paradoxus* may be present, but is usually less marked than in cardiac tamponade.
● *Heart size*. Clinically the heart is usually of normal size or only slightly enlarged. Due to adhesions from the pericardium to the chest wall, in about half the cases there is systolic indrawing of the anterior chest wall.
● *Other features of the condition are generally similar to those of cardiac tamponade*
a   *A small volume pulse* with sinus tachycardia as the heart attempts to maintain cardiac output. However, in about a third of the cases the pulse is irregular due to atrial fibrillation.
b   *A markedly raised jugular venous pulse* often with prominent x and y descents, and sometimes with a paradoxical increase on inspiration (Kussmaul's sign).
c   *The heart sounds* may be quiet and distant, but in contrast to cardiac tamponade often there is a third heart sound.

19   Other organs affected by chronic constrictive pericarditis

● *Liver and spleen*. Jaundice, hepatomegaly and splenomegaly sometimes occur as a result of venous congestion.
● *Kidney and gut*. Occasionally the nephrotic syndrome or protein losing enteropathy occurs as a result of venous congestion.

20   The investigation of chronic constrictive pericarditis

● *ECG*. This usually shows either sinus tachycardia or atrial fibrillation. The voltage is often low and there may be flattening or inversion of the T wave.
● *Chest x-ray*. The heart size is usually normal or only slightly increased. In about half the cases pericardial calcification may be seen, particularly on a lateral film or with cardiac screening. The lung fields are usually clear.
● *Echocardiogram*. Frequently this is unhelpful, although pericardial fluid or thickening may be observed.
● *Cardiac catheterisation*. Characteristically in chronic constrictive pericarditis the end diastolic pressure within each of the four chambers of the heart is the same to within 5 mmHg. In addition catheterisation may allow demonstration of the thickened pericardium.

21   Treatment of chronic constrictive pericarditis

This is by pericardotomy. Before operation diuretics may be given cautiously, taking care not to drastically reduce the high venous pressure required to maintain cardiac output.

22   The differential diagnosis of ascites

Reduced plasma oncotic pressure due to hypoalbuminaemia resulting from:

● *Deficient intake of protein* due for example to starvation or malabsorption.
● *Failure to produce albumin* due to liver disease such as cirrhosis.
● *Abnormal loss of albumin via:*
a   The *kidney* due to nephrotic syndrome.
b   The *gut* due to protein losing enteropathy.
c   The *skin* due to pemphigus or exfoliative dermatitis.

Increased hepatic venous pressure due to:

● Right heart failure.
● Chronic constrictive pericarditis.
● Budd–Chiari syndrome (thrombosis of the hepatic veins).

Increased portal vein pressure

● This may be due to cirrhosis of the liver. Other factors

contributing to the ascites in this situation are hypoproteinaemia and sodium retention.

Increased permeability of the peritoneal capillaries to albumin due to:

- Malignancy involving the peritoneum.
- Infection of the peritoneum, due for example to:
  Tuberculosis.
  Pyogenic peritonitis.

Lymphatic obstruction

This is rare and is due to obstruction of the thoracic duct or mesenteric lymph nodes, usually by tumour.

Metabolic

- This is a rare manifestation of hypothyroidism.

Comment

The importance of recognising the symptoms and signs of chronic constrictive pericarditis is amply demonstrated by the following case.

For about a year, Mr S-A, a 68 year old retired hotelier, had noticed gross swelling of the abdomen which he had been told was due to ascites. However, as he felt reasonably well he did not pursue the matter. When he eventually presented he said that despite fluid retention due to the ascites he had lost 24 lb in weight, and complained that his arms and legs had become very thin. On direct questioning he admitted to slight breathlessness on exertion, but denied any swelling of the ankles or chest pain. There was no past history of tuberculosis and although he had been a hotelier he insisted that he had never taken more than 10 alcoholic drinks per week.

Initially, the diagnosis seemed obscure. Hypoproteinaemia seemed unlikely as there was only the merest trace of protein in the urine, liver function tests were normal, and in any case his serum albumin was normal. Sampling of the peritoneal fluid for malignant cells was negative.

The correct diagnosis was suggested by finding that the jugular venous pulse was elevated to the ears with a slight paradoxical increase on inspiration (Kussmaul's sign), and that the blood pressure showed arterial pulsus paradoxus 10–15 mmHg. Subsequently a chest x-ray showed pericardial calcification.

Following pericardotomy Mr S-A's symptoms and signs all resolved.

Further Reading

Braunwald E (ed) (1984). *Heart Disease*, 2nd edition. WB Saunders, Philadelphia. Chapter 41, diseases of the pericardium.

Case G **A Case of High Blood Pressure: Mr R-C, aged 28 years**

A happily married television repair engineer living with his wife and son in a rented corporation house.

History of present condition

A symptomless young man admitted to hospital for assessment of blood pressure found to be 250/140 during a medical examination for an insurance policy.

Past medical history and family history

Nil of note.

Relevant direct questions

A non-smoker. No history of headache, dizziness, chest pain, breathlessness, swelling of the ankles or palpitations.

Examination

Well looking anxious young man in whom clinical examination was normal except for a sustained apex beat displaced to the anterior axillary line, and an abnormally loud second heart sound in the aortic area. Fundoscopy revealed arteriolar narrowing, an increased light reflex ('silver wiring') and tortuosity of the fundal arteries. On the ward the blood pressure was persistently 180–200/120–140 during the period before treatment was commenced.

Mr R-C

Questions

1   What is unusual about this case? To what should it alert you?
2   Put on your 'hypertension hat' and list the special features of the examination of every hypertensive patient that help to exclude a secondary or treatable cause of the condition.

Answers

1   Unusual feature of the case

The patient's age is the unusual feature of this case. *Primary or essential* hypertension for which the cause is unknown may occur at any age. In patients aged over 35–40 hypertension is invariably of this type. By contrast, about a fifth of patients aged less than 35–

40 have hypertension of the *secondary* type for which a cause that is sometimes reversible may be found. For this reason patients under age 35–40 should be investigated along the lines described later in this chapter. In Mr R-C's case this led to the discovery of stenosis of the right renal artery that was treated with balloon angioplasty, the blood pressure subsequently falling to 140/80 mmHg.

2   The special features of the examination of every hypertensive patient that help to exclude a secondary or treatable cause of the condition

● The appearance of the patient	?Cushingoid or acromegalic appearance
● Palpation of the kidneys	?Enlarged polycystic or hydronephrotic kidneys
● Auscultation of the upper abdomen	?Renal bruit suggesting renal artery stenosis*
● Simultaneous palpation of the radial and femoral or foot arteries	?Delay or absence of the femoral pulse suggesting coarctation of the aorta

* A bruit was audible over Mr R-C's right hypochondrium. However, it is important to appreciate that the specificity and sensitivity of this sign are low, bruits often being heard in normotensive people, particularly young women and the elderly, and in only about 50% of patients with renal artery stenosis.

Chapter 9
Systemic Hypertension

Physiology of the blood pressure; definition of hypertension

Questions

1i What are the two main physiological factors that determine blood pressure? What is the main haemodynamic abnormality in most cases of hypertension?

ii What are the main factors determining systolic pressure?

iii What is the main factor determining diastolic pressure?

2 With regard to using a sphygmomanometer, what are the sounds used to define the systolic and the diastolic blood pressures? What are the Korotkoff sounds?

3 At what times of the day is the blood pressure usually at its lowest and at its highest levels?

4 Which is the more important prognostic index of future adverse cardiovascular events, systolic or diastolic blood pressure?

5 What are the three or four factors that make it difficult to give a precise definition of the term hypertension? Having considered them, attempt to define hypertension.

Answers

1   The factors determining blood pressure

i   *The two main physiological factors.* Blood pressure depends upon the multiple of cardiac output × peripheral resistance. Each of these parameters is in turn dependent upon other factors. Cardiac output is the multiple of stroke volume and pulse rate, and as stated on page 28, stroke volume depends upon the filling pressure of the heart (preload), the intrinsic contractility of the heart muscle, and the load against which the heart has to pump (afterload). In its turn preload is affected by the volume of fluid in the circulation.

Peripheral resistance is determined to a large extent by the width of the lumen of the arterioles, and is discussed on page 163.

●   *In the great majority of patients with established hypertension the main haemodynamic abnormality is an increase of peripheral resistance. By contrast, cardiac output is normal or slightly reduced*, although in a few cases it is increased initially.

ii   *The main factors determining systolic pressure* are the volume of blood ejected during systole, and the response to it or the compliance or elasticity of the walls of the arterial tree. If the stroke volume is small, or alternatively if the arterial walls are very distensible, the systolic pressure will be low. If the stroke volume is large or the walls of the vessels are rigid, the systolic pressure will be high.

iii   *Diastolic pressure is determined* mainly by the elasticity of the arterial walls, gripping and exerting pressure upon the blood whilst the aortic valve is closed and the heart is not pumping. Diastolic pressure ensures a flow of blood during diastole as well as systole and is responsible for filling of the coronary arteries during diastole.

2   The sounds used to define the systolic and the diastolic blood pressures with a sphygmomanometer. The Korotkoff sounds

As the column of mercury is lowered, the *systolic* blood pressure is the reading at which a distinct tapping sound is first heard in time with the pulse. This is the first phase described by Korotkoff.

The *diastolic* pressure is the reading at which the tapping *disappears*, and is the fifth phase described by Korotkoff.

The fourth phase described by Korotkoff is the pressure at which the tapping sounds become *muffled*. Comparison with directly measured intra-arterial pressures shows that the fifth phase or pressure at which the sound disappears is closer to the true diastolic pressure than the fourth phase, which is why the fifth phase is preferred.

3   The times of day at which the blood pressure is generally at its lowest and highest levels

Shortlived changes of blood pressure occur throughout the day in response to activity and emotion. Although it rarely shows with readings taken by a sphygmomanometer, continuous intra-arterial pressure recordings reveal that in both normotensive and hypertensive people the blood pressure shows a diurnal variation, being lowest in the early part of the night and highest in the hour or so before waking in the morning. In hypertensives the diurnal variation is exaggerated.

4   Systolic and diastolic blood pressures as prognostic indices of future adverse cardiovascular events

It is often stated that systolic blood pressure is a better prognostic indicator than diastolic pressure. However, several large surveys suggest that diastolic pressure is a better predictor of adverse events in persons aged under 45, and that systolic pressure, reflecting rigidity and lack of compliance of the arteries, is a better prognostic indicator in persons aged over sixty. Between ages 45 and 60 systolic and diastolic pressures have about the same predictive power.

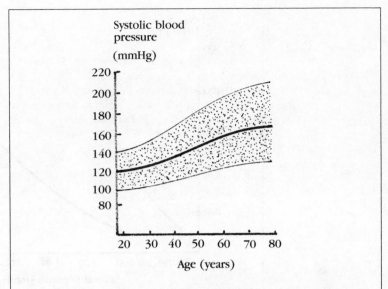

Figure 44. Scatter of systolic blood pressure at any age, and increase of systolic blood pressure with age in an adult population (after Boe)

5   The factors that make it difficult to give a precise definition of the term hypertension, and an attempted definition

Many textbooks state that in practical terms hypertension is a sustained blood pressure above 140/90 mmHg. However, this is an over simplification for the following reasons:

●   As Figure 44 shows, in Western societies the average blood pressure of apparently healthy persons increases with age indicating that it is fallacious to choose any one blood pressure as normal or abnormal for all ages.

●   As Figure 44 also shows, at any particular age in such a society there is a scatter of blood pressures among apparently healthy people.

●   As Figure 45 shows, the risk of adverse cardiovascular events is a continuum with no cut off level beneath which diseases related to the height of the blood pressure do not occur. From the lowest so-called normal levels of blood pressure the risk of cardiovascular events such as a stroke, heart failure and myocardial infarction increases as the blood pressure increases.

However, at any age there is no doubt that a high blood pressure carries a greater risk of adverse events than a low blood pressure. Based on the concept of the increased risk that it implies, *probably the best definition of hypertension is that it is a sustained blood pressure above the average for the person's age.*

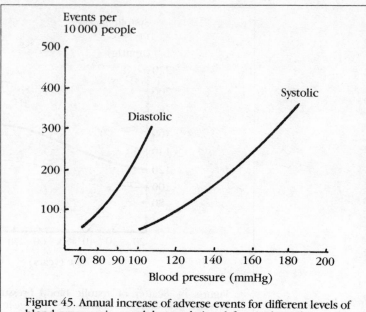

Figure 45. Annual increase of adverse events for different levels of blood pressure in an adult population (after Anderson)

The different forms of hypertension

Questions

6   Define the terms:
i   Essential hypertension. What percentage of hypertensive patients fall into this category?
ii   Secondary hypertension. What percentage of hyptertensives fall into this category? List its causes; which of them are treatable or potentially treatable?
iii Malignant hypertension. What symptoms often accompany this form of hypertension?
iv   Labile hypertension.
7   What is systolic hypertension? What are its main causes?

Answers

6   **Definitions and comments upon the terms**

i   *Essential hypertension*. This is the term applied to hypertension for which the cause is currently unknown. It may not be a single entity, but may have several aetiologies resulting, as previously stated, in an increase of peripheral resistance. Hypotheses regarding the cause of essential hypertension are discussed in the answer to question 8. Over 95% of hypertensives fall into this category.

ii   *Secondary hypertension* is hypertension secondary to a specific identifiable cause. Less than 5% of hypertensives fall into this category. Secondary hypertension is more likely in persons aged under 30–40. Its importance lies in the fact that in some cases the cause is reversible, offering the chance of curing the hypertension. For this reason the possibility of secondary hypertension must be considered in every hypertensive patient. The causes of secondary hypertension:

Endocrine

- Acromegaly*
- Phaeochromocytoma*

Due to salt and water retention

- Cushing's disease*
- Steroid therapy*
- Primary aldosteronism*
- Oral contraceptive*
- Carbenoxolone*

Renal disease

- Chronic glomerulonephritis
- Chronic pyelonephritis
- Polycystic disease
- Renin producing carcinoma*
- Obstructive uropathy*
- Analgesic nephropathy*
- Renal stones*

Vascular

- Renal artery stenosis*
- Coarctation of the aorta*

* Treatable or potentially treatable conditions.

iii   *Malignant hypertension (also known as accelerated hypertension)* is defined as severe hypertension associated with haemorrhages, exudates and sometimes papilloedema in the fundi. It may occur with either essential or secondary hypertension, and is usually associated with diastolic pressures greater than 120 mmHg. The importance of malignant hypertension lies in the fact that without treatment it carries a very poor prognosis with a one year mortality of 95%, usually from cardiac and/or renal failure. It is associated with particular pathological changes in the arterioles that are discussed on page 164.

The symptoms that may occur with malignant hypertension are morning occipital headache, blurred vision due to the retinopathy, breathlessness due to stiffness or failure of the left ventricle, and in the presence of renal failure, symptoms of uraemia.

iv   *Labile hypertension* is the term used to describe hypertension associated with blood pressure readings that are more variable than those usually found. Some authorities believe that labile hypertension is not a discrete entity, but merely represents the changes of blood pressure that occur in all of us, normotensives and hypertensives, throughout the day with emotion, exercise and the cold.

Labile blood pressure is the term used to describe blood pressure that is normal at times and abnormally high at other times. Some authorities believe labile blood pressure is a risk factor for the later development of sustained hypertension.

From a practical point of view the importance of labile hypertension and labile blood pressure is that they make assessment of the blood pressure difficult.

7   Systolic hypertension

This is a sustained elevation of systolic blood pressure above the average for a person's age. Systolic hypertension occurs in conditions in which the stroke volume is relatively large compared with the capacity of the arterial tree. This results in relative overfilling of the arterial system during systole. Systolic hypertension is caused by:

- *Lack of elasticity and compliance* of the arteries in the elderly.
- *Conditions in which the stroke volume is increased*, for example aortic regurgitation, anaemia, thyrotoxicosis, anxiety, fever.

Aetiology of essential hypertension
Question

8   The cause of essential hypertension is unknown. Write a few lines about each of the following aetiological factors that have been suggested as possible causes of the condition:
i   Genetic disposition
ii   Salt intake
iii   Overactivity of the sympathetic nervous system
iv   Baroreceptor insensitivity
v   The kidney and fluid volume control
vi   The renin-angiotensin system
vii   Other factors such as natiuretic hormone and snoring

Answer

8   Suggested aetiological factors in the causation of essential hypertension

The observation has already been made that essential hypertension may not be a single entity, but may have several aetiologies. Among the aetiological factors suggested are:

i   *Genetic disposition*. This is suggested by the occurrence of hypertension in families. It is also suggested by the fact that patients with essential hypertension and their relatives, but not patients with secondary hypertension, have a defect of sodium efflux from their cells resulting in abnormally high levels of intracellular sodium. The significance of this is not understood, although as explained on page 45 it is possible that it may result in an increase of intracellular calcium that in its turn may increase the contractility of arteriolar smooth muscle causing an increase of peripheral resistance and hypertension.

ii   *Salt intake*. Although extreme restriction of salt to about 10 mmoles per day results in significant lowering of the blood pressure, moderate salt restriction of the type that is acceptable to patients has not been shown to have any useful effect upon raised blood pressure. Similarly, although there is a strong correlation between the salt intake of a population and the prevalence within it of hypertension and its complications, the blood pressure of individual hypertensives is not related to their intake or excretion of salt. Even if lowering the salt intake of the whole population were to lower the average blood pressure by a few millimetres Hg it is not clear that the incidence of hypertension would be altered significantly, although it is possible that an as yet unidentified sub-group of hypertensives are sensitive to salt intake.

iii   *Overactivity of the sympathetic nervous system.* Because acute stress causes blood pressure to rise, it has been suggested that chronic over-stimulation of the sympathetic nervous system by stress may lead to chronic vasoconstriction, an increase of peripheral resistance and hypertension. However, there is considerable overlap between the plasma noradrenaline levels of normotensives and hypertensives, and at the present time the hypothesis is unproven.

iv   *Baroreceptor insensitivity.* A rise of blood pressure stimulates pressure sensitive stretch receptors in the carotid sinus and aortic arch to discharge impulses that inhibit the outflow of sympathetic impulses from the brain to the peripheral arterioles. This results in vasodilatation, decrease in peripheral resistance and a fall in blood pressure. In patients with essential hypertension the sensitivity of the baroreceptors is reduced causing them to respond less vigorously than normal to rises of blood pressure, but whether this is merely a result of damage by the hypertension rather than its cause is not known.

v   *The kidney and control of fluid volume.* Because it controls the amount of salt and water in the body, most authorities feel that the kidney has an important role in the control of blood pressure, but by what mechanism is not clear as the blood volume of most patients with established essential hypertension is normal or low. Our ignorance is exemplified by the fact that we have no real idea as to why only about half the patients with severe diseases of the kidney such as glomerulonephritis and pyelonephritis develop hypertension.

Suggestions have been made that vasoactive substances such as the kinins and prostaglandins acting locally within the kidney may in some way affect its influence upon the blood pressure.

vi   *The renin–angiotensin system.* The enzyme renin is released from the juxta-glomerular apparatus of the kidney when the perfusion pressure in the renal artery falls. As illustrated below, renin acts on the plasma protein, angiotensinogen, to produce angiotensin I which in turn is acted upon by converting enzyme to produce angiotensin II. Together with thromboxane, angiotensin II is one of the most powerful known vasoconstrictors, and in addition also stimulates the release of aldosterone from the adrenal cortex.

Although activation of the renin–angiotensin system is implicated in the hypertension of renal artery stenosis and coarctation of the aorta in which the kidney is underperfused, its role in essential hypertension is doubtful as plasma renin levels are low in about 30% of patients with the condition, are intermediate in about 60%, and are high in only about 10%. Moreover, diuretics have a paradoxical effect, causing blood pressure to fall, and plasma renin levels to rise.

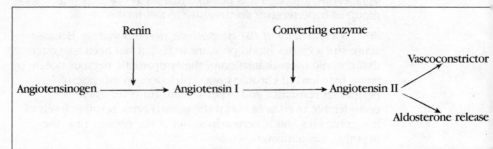

vii   *Other factors*. Atrial natiuretic hormone is a recently isolated hormone that is secreted from the right atrium when that organ is stretched. Its main actions are to cause salt and water loss via the kidney, and vasodilatation. However, its role in hypertension is unclear as some studies report high levels of the hormone in the plasma of hypertensives, whilst others report normal levels.

Regular snoring is also reported to be a risk factor for the development of hypertension, presumably as a result of anoxia causing vasoconstriction.

Pathological effects
Questions

9   Clinically, which organs are most commonly affected by hypertension? List the clinical syndromes that may affect each organ as a result of hypertension.

10i   What are the main histological effects of hypertension upon medium sized arteries such as the radial artery, and what are the main histological effects of (a) essential hypertension, and (b) malignant hypertension upon the smaller arteries and arterioles?

ii   What are the main effects of hypertension upon the histology of the heart?

iii   What are Charcot-Bouchard aneurysms?

iv   Apart from its effects upon the vasculature, what are the other main histological effects of hypertension upon the kidney?

Answers

9 The organs most commonly affected by hypertension and the resulting clinical syndromes and effects

Organ	Clinical effect
The arteries	● Narrowing and an increase of peripheral resistance. The mechanism underlying this is described in the answer to the next question ● In the brain, rupture may result in cerebral haemorrhage
The heart	● Angina of effort ● Myocardial infarction ● Left ventricular failure
The brain	● Stroke due to accelerated atherosclerosis ● Stroke due to cerebral haemorrhage ● Transient ischaemic attack (TIA) ● Hypertensive encephalopathy
The eye	● Hypertensive retinopathy—discussed in the answer to question 14 ● Clinically the changes associated with malignant hypertension may cause blurring of vision
The kidney	● Mild hypertension usually has little functional effect upon the kidney. Severe hypertension may cause proteinuria, microscopic or macroscopic haematuria, and renal failure

10 The main histological effects of hypertension upon the arteries, heart and kidneys

i *Medium sized arteries:* hypertension is associated with two main changes in the walls of the medium sized arteries such as the radial artery, both of which lead to narrowing of the lumen of the vessel and an increase of peripheral resistance. These changes are:
● Thickening of the media and intima.
● Accelerated atherosclerosis.
Small arteries and arterioles: in addition to accelerated atherosclerosis, hypertension may cause the following specific changes:

(a) *Essential hypertension.* Especially in the small arteries and arterioles of the kidney, and to a lesser extent the brain and mesentery, but only occasionally in muscle, essential hypertension is associated with:

- *The deposition of hyaline* due, it is thought, to plasma proteins and lipids being forced into the vessel wall.
- *Reduplication of the elastic lamina* of the vessel wall.

(b)   *Malignant hypertension.* In the small arteries and arterioles of the same tissues malignant hypertension causes:

- *Fibrinoid neocrosis*—the deposition of a substance similar to fibrin, often in association with an inflammatory infiltrate.
- *Onion skinning*—reduplication of the smooth muscle of the arterial wall.

ii   *The heart.* As explained on page 31 hypertension is often associated with hypertrophy of the muscle cells of the heart. If as a consequence the heart 'outgrows' its blood supply or the walls of the coronary arteries become narrowed, the muscle fibres may become relatively ischaemic and degenerate, resulting in patchy fibrosis.

iii   *Charcot-Bouchard aneurysms.* These are microaneurysms up to about 1 mm in diameter in the small arteries of the brain of hypertensive people but not normotensives, and were described by Charcot and Bouchard in the striate arteries of the base of the brain approximately 100 years ago. Rupture of Charcot-Bouchard aneurysms is probably a major cause of cerebral haemorrhage.

iv   *The kidney.* Apart from the changes described above in the small arteries and arterioles of the kidney, hypertension is associated with sclerosis of glomeruli, tubular atrophy and fibrosis of the interstitium.

Symptoms and signs
Questions

11   What symptoms are associated with hypertension?
12   What is hypertensive encephalopathy; to what is it thought to be due?
13   What signs are associated with hypertension? (Note that the retinal changes are the subject of the next question.)
14i   Describe the various grades of hypertensive retinopathy.
    ii   What is the mechanism by which each of the changes is thought to occur?

Answers

11   The symptoms of hypertension

Usually hypertension is a symptomless finding. Except for the morning occipital headache of malignant hypertension, headache is no more common in hypertensive than normotensive people. If organ damage has occurred symptoms related to the clinical syndromes listed on page 163 may occur.

12 Hypertensive encephalopathy

This is an unusual life threatening complication of severe hypertension and is associated with the development of central nervous symptoms such as drowsiness, confusion, dysphasia, minor strokes or fits. Hypertensive encephalopathy may occur with or without the retinal changes of malignant hypertension. Usually the diastolic pressure is higher than 120 mmHg, but occasionally may be as low as 110 mmHg. Hypertensive encephalopathy is associated with *focal swelling* of the brain most probably due to leakage of plasma from damaged arterioles and capillaries. It is an indication for rapid lowering of the blood pressure.

13 The signs associated with hypertension

Apart from examining the patient for causes of secondary hypertension such as renal artery stenosis, coarctation of the aorta and polycystic or hydronephrotic kidneys, the main features of the examination in hypertension are to assess organ damage. Hypertension may give the pulse a hard atherosclerotic quality and cause retinopathy, and as described below may also cause changes in the heart sounds and cardiomegaly.

Nonetheless, in most cases there are no specific signs. When signs are present, among the commoner the aortic component of the second heart sound (A2) is often louder than normal over the aortic or second right intercostal space. Non-significant systolic flow murmurs are sometimes audible. A fourth sound reflecting stiffness of the left ventricle may also be heard.

If the heart has hypertrophied sufficiently the apex beat may be sustained and displaced laterally, and very occasionally splitting of the second heart sound may be reversed or paradoxical (see page 18).

14 Hypertensive retinopathy: clinical manifestations and mechanisms

i Hypertensive retinopathy is divided into four grades. Grades I and II are associated with mild/moderate hypertension; grades III and IV with malignant hypertension. Because the prognosis with modern treatment is the same for patients with grades III and IV retinopathy it has been suggested that the division of these grades is artificial. Description of the grades is as follows:

Grade	Description
I	• Arterial narrowing • Increased light reflex (silver wiring)
II	• Arteriolar-venous (A-V) nipping and tortuosity of the arteries
III	• Soft or cotton wool exudates • Haemorrhages
IV	• Papilloedema • Hard exudates fanning out from the macula, usually developing after papilloedema

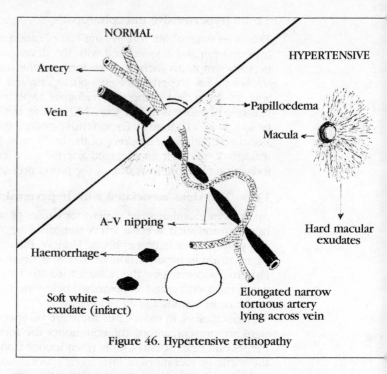

Figure 46. Hypertensive retinopathy

ii   Mechanisms of retinopathy:

•   *Grades I and II*. Arterial narrowing is due to spasm of the muscle in the arterial wall. The increased light reflex, tortuosity and A-V nipping are due to thickening and lengthening of the arterial wall and may occur in atherosclerosis as well as hypertension, and as a consequence are non-specific signs in the elderly. In particular, the increased light reflex is due to light being reflected back from the thickened wall of the artery in contrast to the normal situation in which the wall is transparent and transmits light through to the red blood cells within. Similarly A-V nipping is due to elongated arteries twisting to lie upon their accompanying veins.

•   *Grades III and IV*. The changes associated with these grades are due either to *ischaemia or abnormal permeability* of the retinal arteries and capillaries. Thus soft or cotton wool exudates are due to disruption and debris from damaged nerve fibres as a result of *ischaemia*, and haemorrhages to *leakage* of red blood cells, papilloedema to *leakage* of plasma, and the hard exudates around the macula to *leakage* and deposition of lipids within the deeper layers of the retina.

Investigation
Questions

15   List the specific investigations that should be performed in a case of essential hypertension. Describe your reasons for ordering the tests and the abnormalities you would be looking for.

16 In which hypertensive patients is it generally agreed that further investigation is justified in an effort to find a treatable underlying cause of the hypertension?

17 Briefly describe the pathological causes of each of the following conditions, and the tests that may be ordered in their investigation: (i) renal artery stenosis, (ii) phaeochromocytoma, (iii) mineralocorticoid excess, (iv) coarctation of the aorta.

Answers

15 The specific investigation of a case of essential hypertension

- *Testing the urine*. The presence of proteinura, haematuria and cell casts indicates renal damage.
- *Serum creatinine or urea* to assess renal function and any effect of the hypertension upon it.
- *Serum electrolytes*. Hypokalaemia in a patient not taking diuretics suggests excess mineralocorticoid secretion, for instance primary hyperaldosteronism (Conn's disease).
- *Chest x-ray*. The heart may appear enlarged, but is often normal in size. The aorta may dilate and become elongated and tortuous as a result of the increased pressure within it. Perhaps once in a lifetime rib notching associated with coarctation of the aorta may be seen.
- *Electrocardiogram*. This may be normal or show left axis deviation, left ventricular hypertrophy, 'strain' or pressure overload with ST depression like a tick drawn backwards in the standard and lateral chest leads (see page 39), or the changes of ischaemia (see page 95) or infarction (see page 118).

16 The search for and investigation of treatable underlying causes of hypertension

As has already been discussed on page 158, less than 5% of hypertensive patients have secondary hypertension for which an underlying cause can be identified. In view of this it is generally agreed that further investigation is warranted only in patients in whom the likelihood of finding a secondary cause of their condition is relatively high. Experience has shown these are:
- Patients aged under 40 years.
- Patients with very high blood pressure that is difficult to control.

17 A brief description of the pathological causes and a brief description of the investigation of:

i *Renal artery stenosis*. Narrowing of one or both renal arteries is caused by muscular or fibrous dysplasia of the arterial wall in young persons, particularly young women, and by atheromatous narrowing in the middle-aged and elderly. As a result of the stenosis, the flow of blood into and out of the affected kidney is reduced and delayed, and because of the ischaemia so produced, the kidney on the affected side is usually small and produces excessive amounts of renin.

• *Intravenous pyelography (IVP)* gives information about both the function and anatomy of the kidney, and may show a small kidney and delay in the excretion of contrast medium on the affected side.

• *Isotope renography* gives information about renal blood flow and the excretory function of the kidney, and may show delayed flow of blood into and delayed excretion of isotope from the kidney. However, as both IVP and isotope renography are normal in about 20% of patients with renal artery stenosis, they are usually used as relatively non-invasive screening tests, patients in whom the condition is strongly suspected proceeding to renal arteriography.

• In patients with proven renal artery stenosis comparison of the amounts of renin produced by each kidney, measured by catheterising the renal veins, is often used to assess the likely outcome of surgery. A ratio of 1.5:1 is indicative of likely success, although some patients with a smaller ratio respond to surgery, whilst others with a higher ratio do not, possibly because the other kidney and the blood vessels have been damaged by the hypertension which as a consequence is irreversible without drug therapy.

ii   *Phaeochromocytoma* is due to overproduction of adrenaline and noradrenaline by either a benign or malignant tumour of the adrenal medulla. Phaeochromocytoma should be suspected in hypertensive patients with symptoms of catecholamine overproduction such as pounding headache, palpitations, sweating, agitation, rapid changes of skin colour, and a blood pressure that fluctuates and spikes, although sustained elevation may also occur, whilst due to adrenaline, the blood pressure may even be low at times.

In suspected cases elevated levels of the catecholamine metabolites vanillylmandelic acid (VMA) and the metadrenalines are found in the urine. Plasma catecholamine levels are also elevated.

iii   *Mineralocorticoid overproduction* is usually due to an adenoma or bilateral hyperplasia of the adrenal cortex. In most patients the condition is suggested by finding hypokalaemia in the absence of diuretic therapy. Further investigations show elevated plasma levels of aldosterone, and as a result of this, depressed plasma renin levels.

iv   *Coarctation of the aorta* is due to a narrowing of the thoracic aorta, in the adult usually just below the origin of the left subclavian artery. The condition is fully discussed on page 198.

It may lead to hypertension in the upper half of the body. The cause of hypertension is unknown, but may be due to the increased systolic tension developed by the left ventricle in response to the obstruction, or to activation of the angiotensin-renin system in the ischaemic lower half of the body, or both. In those with delayed or absent femoral pulses, the investigation of choice is an aortogram.

Assessment; when and why to treat

Questions

18 What proportion of hypertensives are likely to be receiving adequate treatment?

19i How long a period of observation is generally recommended before beginning the drug treatment of hypertension?

ii What is the likelihood that the blood pressure of a person with suspected mild hypertension will revert spontaneously to normal?

iii Which conditions or complications of hypertension occur less frequently with adequate treatment, and which occur as frequently or almost as frequently despite treatment?

iv Approximately how many patients with mild hypertension, diastolic pressure at the commencement of treatment 90-110 mmHg, must be treated for a year in order to prevent one stroke? Above what sustained level of blood pressure do most authorities recommend that drug treatment should be given?

Answers

18 The proportion of hypertensives likely to be receiving adequate treatment

Surveys have shown that the proportion of hypertensives likely to be receiving adequate treatment is surprisingly small. The size of the challenge is best expressed by the 'rule of fours' which implies that for every adequately treated hypertensive there is a second who is inadequately treated, a third who is known to the medical profession but not receiving any treatment, and a fourth who is not even known to the medical profession.

19 Assessment of the blood pressure before treatment, and the likely results of treatment

i Treatment should be commenced with the first high blood pressure reading in patients with clear evidence of organ damage, such as marked cardiomegaly, ECG evidence of 'strain' or pressure overload, or grades III or IV retinopathy.

In patients without evidence of organ damage several readings should be taken over a period of 2 or 3 weeks or even months with the patient lying comfortably relaxed to make sure that any high readings obtained are sustained and are not merely a temporary phenomenon due to anxiety.

ii The need for caution in making a diagnosis on the basis of a few readings is reflected by the fact that the blood pressure spontaneously reverts to normal in about a third of patients thought to have mild symptomless hypertension, defined as diastolic pressure 90-110 mmHg on at least three occasions. Indeed it has been said that casual mild elevations of the blood pressure are about as non-specific as temperature in predicting patient outcome or indicating a need for treatment. For this reason some authorities recommend observing the blood pressure of such patients for up to 6 months before deciding about treatment.

iii   Reducing the blood pressure of a hypertensive patient reduces the likelihood of stroke, transient ischaemic attack, heart failure and renal failure, but has little or no effect upon the likelihood of myocardial infarction, which numerically is by far the most common condition. However, treatment may reduce the incidence of myocardial infarction in two subgroups, namely the elderly, and also non-smoking males treated with beta blocking drugs.

iv   Trials have shown a clear benefit for the treatment of patients with sustained diastolic pressures above about 110 mmHg, but for pressures below this, in the range of 90–110 mmHg any benefits are rather marginal. Thus even with a condition such as stroke that is rendered less likely with treatment, it is necessary to treat no fewer than 850 patients in this range for a year in order to prevent one stroke.

Faced with the need to balance the benefits of treatment against the side effects of the available drugs, and the not inconsiderable dilemma of turning people who feel healthy into patients, it is generally agreed that the blood pressure above which treatment is indicated is a sustained diastolic pressure of 100 mmHg or more. At the present time few doctors treat lone systolic hypertension, probably mainly from a wish not to lower a normal diastolic pressure to abnormally low and possibly hazardous levels.

How much to lower the pressure; the elderly; stopping treatment
Question

20i   To what levels is it recommended that the blood pressure should be lowered?

ii   Up to what age do elderly patients probably benefit from treatment?

iii   What is the likely result of stopping treatment in patients in whom treatment has been associated with years of 'normalised' blood pressure, say 140/85?

Answer

20i   The diastolic pressure should probably be reduced to no lower than 85–90 mmHg as this appears to be the level at which the greatest benefit is obtained and the incidence of the complications of hypertension is least. Filling of the coronary arteries occurs in diastole, and it has been suggested, but is disputed, that the reason that the treatment of hypertension has failed to lower the incidence of myocardial infarction is that in many cases the diastolic pressure and filling of the coronary arteries in diastole have been lowered too much.

ii   A large trial has shown that the elderly benefit from the treatment of hypertension up to the age of about 80, although in practice, for fear of side effects, most physicians tend to be cautious about the treatment of persons aged over 70-75 years.

iii   Although it may be tempting to stop hypertensive treatment in patients whose blood pressure has been 'normal' for several years, several studies have shown that over a period of months the blood pressure rises to hypertensive levels in about 90% of patients in whom treatment is stopped. The moral is therefore to resist the temptation of stopping the treatment of patients whose hypertension was well authenticated to begin with.

How to treat hypertension
Questions

21   What is the main aim of the treatment of hypertension? By what general principles is it achieved?

22   The increased morbidity and mortality of hypertension is compounded by many other important risk factors, some of which like alcohol intake are potentially reversible, whilst others like the sex of the patient are not. Prepare a list of these prognostic risk factors to help you assess and advise your hypertensive patients.

23   List the various types or classes of drugs used in the modern treatment of hypertension. What are their modes of action and main side effects?

24   By how much on average do recommended doses of each class of drug lower the systolic and diastolic pressures?

Answers

21   The main aim of the treatment of hypertension and the principles by which it is achieved

The main aim of the treatment of hypertension is to reduce the likelihood of any of the complications of raised blood pressure. This is achieved by:

● Careful assessment of the patient and the need for treatment.

● Identification, and where possible, rectification of the causes of secondary hypertension.

● Modification of the risk factors discussed in the answer to the next question.

● Reduction of the blood pressure.

22   The risk factors other than high blood pressure that contribute to the morbidity and mortality of hypertension

Addressing the other risk factors that are reversible is often as important as lowering the blood pressure, although in the interests of patient co-operation it is probably best to proceed gently, addressing one at a time.

Figure 47 shows the importance of some of these factors, which are:

● *Sex of the patient.* Women tolerate and suffer less morbidity and mortality from a raised blood pressure than men.

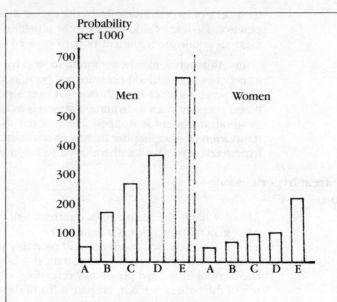

A = cholesterol 185mg%
B = cholesterol 335mg%
C = cholesterol 335mg% + glucose intolerance
D = cholesterol 335mg% + glucose intolerance + cigarette smoking
E = cholesterol 335mg% + glucose intolerance + cigarette smoking
    + ECG LVH

Figure 47.
Systolic blood pressure 150 mmHg: 8 year risk of cardiovascular
event according to other risk factors. Framingham study

- *Height of the blood pressure*. Figure 45 shows that the risk
of adverse events is related to the height of both the systolic and
diastolic pressures.
- *State of the arteries*. For instance, without treatment, grades
III and IV retinopathy carry 95% one year mortality.

- *Cigarette smoking*	Hypertension increases the
- *Obesity*	risk of ischaemic heart
- *Elevation of plasma lipids*	disease. The main effect of
- *Glucose intolerance*	each of these factors is to add
	to that risk.

- *Alcohol*. In both normotensives and hypertensives the regular
consumption of as little as three alcoholic drinks per day raises the
blood pressure by about 5-9 mmHg, an effect that is rapidly
reversed within a week or so of stopping alcohol. Overall it has
been estimated that alcohol consumption accounts for about 10–
30% of essential hypertension.

- Left ventricular	The function of the heart and
hypertrophy (LVH)	the kidney usually improves
- Renal impairment	with appropriate treatment.

23 The various classes of drugs used in the treatment of hypertension, their modes of action and main side effects

● *Thiazide diuretics*. These have a greater hypotensive effect than the loop diuretics. In hypertension their action appears to be in two phases, an initial phase related to reduction of plasma volume, and a long-term phase related to a reduction of peripheral resistance, possibly as a result of intracellular fluid and electrolyte changes causing reduced contractility of the smooth muscle cells of the arterial wall.

The side effects of the thiazide diuretics are discussed on page 44.

● *Beta blocking drugs*. The actions and side effects of these drugs are discussed on page 100.

Labetalol has both alpha and ß adrenergic blocking effects, and is particularly useful in patients with renal failure as it is largely metabolised and excreted by the liver.

● *Vasodilators*. These drugs act by reducing peripheral resistance. Examples are:

a *The calcium antagonists* nifedipine and verapamil. The actions and side effects of these drugs are discussed on page 101.

b *Hydrallazine*. This drug acts by directly relaxing vascular smooth muscle. Its main side effects are reflex tachycardia, and drug induced systemic lupus erythematosus.

c *Prazosin*. This drug competitively inhibits post-synaptic alpha$_1$, adrenoreceptors. Its main side effect is occasional severe hypotension with the first dose of the drug.

d *Angiotensin converting enzyme inhibitors (ACE inhibitors)* such as captopril and enalapril. The action of these drugs is to inhibit the conversion of angiotensin I to angiotensin II, and also to suppress the secretion of aldosterone and inhibit the synthesis of kinins.

e *Other drugs* used occasionally include minoxidil which acts by directly relaxing vascular smooth muscle. The main side effects of minoxidil are fluid retention and hirsutism that usually makes the drug unacceptable to women.

NOTE: Drugs such as guanethidine, debrisoquine, reserpine, clonidine and methyldopa are no longer generally used, although methyldopa is still a standard drug for the treatment of pregnancy related hypertension.

24 Effect of drugs on blood pressure levels

On average, recommended doses of each of the various types of drug lower the diastolic pressure by about 5-15 mmHg, and systolic pressure by about 10-25 mmHg.

Order of using the drugs; rapid lowering of the blood pressure
Questions

25 In the answer to question 23 you were asked to list the various classes of drugs used in the modern treatment of hypertension. Now suggest the order in which you would use each

of the classes of drug in the outpatient treatment of hypertension, that is

i   With which types of drug would you begin treatment?

ii   What would you do if the drug you chose to start with proved insufficient?

iii   Which are the third line drugs? When are they used?

26i   What are the indications for rapid lowering of the blood pressure in hypertension?

ii   Which drugs are usually used to accomplish it safely?

Answers

25   The order in which the various classes of hypotensive drugs are usually used

i   Prescribing is largely a matter of habit and of balancing the efficacy and side effects of established drugs against the efficacy and side effects of new drugs. Competent treatment is probably best achieved by becoming familiar with and sticking to one or two drugs from each of the modern groups of medication.

At the present time it is usual to begin treatment with either a thiazide diuretic or a beta blocking drug. Despite various theoretical considerations, the efficacy and overall safety of both groups of drugs is about the same. Which to choose is therefore somewhat arbitrary but may be helped by the following considerations. As it is less likely to cause impotence, a beta blocker is probably preferable in sexually active males, particularly those who do not smoke in whom such drugs have a cardioprotective effect. Because of their action in angina, a beta blocker is also preferable in patients with both angina due to ischaemic heart disease and hypertension. On the other hand beta blocking drugs are contraindicated in patients with asthma, chronic obstructive airways disease and heart failure, and are relatively contraindicated in patients with peripheral vascular disease.

ii   First remember that most hypotensive drugs take up to 3 weeks to have their full effect. If after that time, or before if the blood pressure remains very high, the beta blocker or thiazide diuretic you have chosen is not working, add the other, that is add a beta blocker to a thiazide, or vice versa.

iii   If the combination of a beta blocker and a thiazide proves insufficient, or is contraindicated, it is usual to incorporate third line therapy, for example:

●   Add nifedipine, hydrallazine or prazosin

●   Change to gradually increasing doses of captopril or enalapril ± thiazide diuretic

●   Change to verapamil ± thiazide diuretic

26   The indications for rapid lowering of blood pressure and the drugs used to achieve it safely

i   Lowering the blood pressure rapidly over a period of *minutes* is potentially dangerous and should be avoided as it may cause cerebral ischaemia, prolonged unconsciousness and neurological damage. In hypertensive encephalopathy, and severe left ventricular failure secondary to hypertension, the blood pressure should be lowered smoothly over *an hour or so*; in malignant hypertension this period should probably be extended to a few days.

In the case of left ventricular failure it should be appreciated that rather than reflecting true sustained hypertension, sometimes a raised blood pressure reflects a temporary reflex response to impairment of the circulation that will resolve with treatment of the heart failure.

ii   Drugs used to lower blood pressure rapidly and safely are:
● Nifedipine liquid, obtained by biting and swallowing the contents of a 10 mg capsule, repeated as necessary: an easy, safe and relatively rapid way of lowering the blood pressure.
● Hydrallazine, 10–20 mg by slow intravenous injection.
● Diazoxide, 50 mg intravenous boluses, repeated as necessary.

Further Reading

Braunwald E (ed) (1984). *Heart Disease*, 2nd edition. WB
    Saunders, Philadelphia. Chapters 25, systemic hypertension:
    mechanisms and diagnosis; 26, therapy.
Weatherall DJ, Ledingham JGG, Warrell DA (eds) (1987). *Oxford
    Textbook of Medicine*, 2nd edition. Oxford University Press,
    Oxford. Hypertension, pp. 13.360–96.

Case H   # A Case of Joint Pains: Miss J-I, aged 8 years

A schoolgirl living at home with her mother and father and two younger brothers.

History of present condition

A little girl admitted to hospital at the request of her family doctor with a 2 day history of joint pains. Her history began with the development of painful swelling of the right knee, limiting movement. At the same time she felt unwell and lost her appetite. On the following day her right wrist and right elbow became painful. On the day of admission the pain in the right knee resolved, but her left knee became painful, swollen, hot and tender.

Past medical and family history

Nil of note, except for bronchopneumonia aged 4 months.

Drugs on admission

Phenoxymethylpenicillin 250 mg four times per day for one day.

Examination

Pale ill-looking dark haired little girl.
Temperature 38°C. Pulse 100 regular. Respiratory rate 22. Weight 23 kilos.
Examination of the cardiovascular, respiratory and abdominal systems was normal.
Examination of the joints revealed hot tender swellings with limited movement of the right wrist and elbow, right shoulder, and left knee in which there was a large effusion. The right knee was still warm but no longer tender.

Miss J-I
Question

1   List the main differential diagnosis of Miss J-I's condition. What do you think was the most likely diagnosis in her case? What additional piece of history would you have enquired about?

Answer

1   The main differential diagnosis of Miss J-I's condition

- Acute rheumatic fever.
- Juvenile chronic arthritis, including conditions such as juvenile rheumatoid arthritis, juvenile ankylosing spondylitis (unlikely in view of her sex) and Still's disease.
- Septicaemic arthritis, in this age group most probably due to a streptococcus.
- Henoch–Schönlein purpura.
- Reactive arthritis to a viral infection such as mumps.
- Acute leukaemia.

The most likely condition from which Miss J-I was suffering was acute rheumatic fever. Additional enquiry revealed that she had a sore throat 2 weeks prior to admission. The diagnosis of acute rheumatic fever was confirmed by a threefold increase in anti-streptolysin-O titre (ASOT), prolongation of the PR interval on ECG, normal full blood count and negative blood culture. She was treated in the manner discussed in Chapter 10 and made an uneventful recovery.

Chapter 10
Acute Rheumatic Fever

Definition and pathology
Questions

1   Give a definition of acute rheumatic fever. Without treatment, what is the likelihood of a recurrence of the acute condition? What is the likelihood of the condition smouldering on to cause chronic rheumatic heart disease?

2   Describe the immune process by which tissue damage is thought to occur in rheumatic fever. What is an Aschoff nodule?

Answers

1   Definition

Rheumatic fever is an acute disease of the connective tissues, particularly the heart, its valves and the joints, caused by a hyperimmune or autoimmune reaction to an infection in the throat with a Lancefield Group A ß-haemolytic streptococcus.

Apart from its acute effects it is important because of its propensity to recur in up to 70% of cases unless adequate treatment is given, and for its tendency to smoulder on causing chronic rheumatic heart disease later in life in about 50% of patients.

2   Mechanism of tissue damage in acute rheumatic fever

It is thought that the Lancefield Group A ß-haemolytic streptococcus and the patient's connective tissues share common antigens and that the immune reaction mounted by the body against the organism leads to a reaction against the patient's connective tissues causing inflammation, typically with the formation of Aschoff nodules that consist of areas of fibrinoid necrosis surrounded by epithelioid giant cells and an outer layer of lymphocytes.

In about half the cases the condition rumbles on, apparently occultly, causing thickening and distortion of the heart valves that manifests later in life as chronic rheumatic heart disease.

Clinical features
Questions

3i   In what age group is a first attack of rheumatic fever most likely?

ii   What reasons are usually quoted for the decline in the incidence of acute rheumatic fever?

4   The easiest way of thinking about the clinical and laboratory features of acute rheumatic fever is to consider the Jones' criteria for the diagnosis of the acute disease. List the five major and six minor Jones' criteria. How many of each are required for a positive diagnosis? As you make you your list, write notes describing the clinical features of each of the major criteria.

Answers

3   The age of first attack; decline in incidence

i   In the West a first attack is most likely in children aged 7-15, although it may occur outside this age group. In developing countries attacks tend to occur earlier, often in infancy, and are associated with a higher incidence of severe cardiac and valvular disease, and a higher mortality.

ii   Acute rheumatic fever is now rare in the West. Usually this is ascribed to better housing and social conditions and more liberal use of antibiotics resulting in less crowding and less person to person spread of the responsible ß-haemolytic stretococcus. However, recent outbreaks of acute rheumatic fever in the United States suggest that even in affluent societies virulent organisms may cause the disease, and that possibly the organisms in the developed countries have been less virulent in the past few decades.

4   The Jones' criteria for the clinical and laboratory diagnosis of acute rheumatic fever

Acute rheumatic fever usually presents as an acute febrile illness. The Jones' criteria cover most of the clinical and laboratory features of the condition. Two major, or one major and two minor, criteria are required for a positive diagnosis.

The five major criteria

●   *Carditis*. This is suggested by the development of:
a   *Tachycardia* out of proportion to any pyrexia, that is > 20 beats per 1°C fever.
b   *A new apical systolic murmur* due to mitral regurgitation caused by dilatation of the mitral valve ring and failure of the valve cusps to meet.
c   *Carey Coombs murmur*. This is a short mid-diastolic apical murmur due to acute inflammation and swelling of the mitral valve causing an early form of mitral stenosis. The murmur may disappear as the inflammation resolves or develop into the more typical murmur of mitral stenosis.
d   *Cardiac enlargement*, either clinical or on x-ray, due to either true enlargement of the heart or pericardial effusion.
e   *Pericarditis*. This occurs in about 10% of cases and is discussed on page 143.

f   *Frank cardiac failure*. About 10% of cases present this way.
●   *Polyarthritis*. Unlike polyarthralgia, in which joints are painful without objective changes, polyarthritis involves acute inflammation and swelling of the joints, and occurs in about a third of patients with acute rheumatic fever, usually as a flitting painful arthritis of the limb joints that affects large and medium sized joints such as the shoulder, elbow, wrist, hip, knee or ankle joints. After affecting one joint for a day or so, typically the pain and swelling resolve and appear in another joint.
●   *Chorea*. Also known as Sydenham's chorea or St Vitus' dance, this is a rare manifestation of acute rheumatic fever and consists of grimacing and irregular jerky movements in contradistinction to the more writhing movements of athetosis. Generally chorea affects all four limbs, although occasionally only one side is affected when it is known as hemichorea. Chorea is due to the rheumatic process causing inflammation of the brain, and may occur up to 3 or 4 months after the acute illness. It affects girls more than boys, and is often associated with emotional disturbances such as depression, weeping, hysteria and uncontrolled laughter.
●   *Erythema marginatum* is a rare rash consisting of irregular red rings with clear centres on the trunk and proximal parts of the limbs. It is a manifestation of acute hypersensitivity.
●   *Rheumatic nodules*. These are non-tender, palpable inflammatory collections usually about the size of a pea, unattached to the overlying skin.

The six minor criteria

●   Fever.
●   Arthralgia—pain without objective change in a joint.
●   Prolongation of the PR interval on an ECG, > 0.2 msec, indicating delay of conduction between the atria and the ventricles.
●   Elevation of the erythrocyte sedimentation rate (ESR), or C-reactive protein, or a leucocytosis.
●   Evidence of a preceding Lancefield Group A ß-haemolytic streptococcal infection, for instance a positive throat culture or rising anti-streptolysin-O titre (ASOT).
●   Past history of rheumatic fever.

Treatment
Questions

5   Describe how you would treat a case of acute rheumatic fever presenting with:
i   Fever, general unwellness and flitting polyarthritis.
ii   A similar case complicated by carditis with cardiac failure.
iii   Chorea.
6   What prophylaxis should be given against further attacks of rheumatic fever? For how long is it usual to give such prophylaxis?

Answers

5 The treatment of acute rheumatic fever

i   *With fever, unwellness and flitting polyarthritis* the treatment given should be:
- Bed rest, to rest the joints and hopefully reduce the likelihood of carditis.
- Apart from bed rest, other general measures include support of painful joints by pillows, and if necessary of the weight of the bed clothes by a cradle.
- Salicylates, orally every 4 hours for their anti-inflammatory effect with the aim of achieving a therapeutic level of 30–35 mg per litre. The main side effects of large doses of salicylates are nausea, vomiting, tinnitus and deafness. If any of these occur the dose should be reduced.
- Phenoxymethylpenicillin 250 mg four times per day for 5 days, although it should be appreciated that eradicating any streptococci does not alter the course of a current attack of rheumatic fever.

ii   *With carditis and cardiac failure.* In addition to the general measures outlined above, patients with cardiac failure should be given prednisolone 40 mg each morning, together with digitalis and diuretics.

iii   *Chorea* may be controlled with either oral or injected diazepam or a phenothiazine such as chlorpromazine. If chorea occurs as part of the acute illness the measures outlined in section i of this answer should be taken (a) to relieve symptoms and (b) to reduce the likelihood of carditis.

6   Prophylaxis against further attacks of rheumatic fever

Prophylactic phenoxymethylpenicillin 250 mg twice a day, or sulphadimidine 1 gram daily for those who are allergic to penicillin, reduces the rate of recurrence of acute rheumatic fever from 70% to 4%. It is generally agreed that prophylaxis should be taken until at least age 18 years, or for 5 years after an acute attack in older persons.

Further Reading

Braunwald E (ed) (1984). *Heart Disease*, 2nd edition. WB Saunders, Philadelphia. Chapter 47, connective tissue diseases of the cardiovascular system.

Chapter 11
Valvular Disease of the Heart

Chronic rheumatic valvular disease

Questions

1   What is the likelihood of acute rheumatic fever causing chronic rheumatic heart disease in later life? What is the likely interval between an attack of acute rheumatic fever and the onset of symptoms due to chronic rheumatic heart disease?

2   In percentage terms what are the approximate frequencies with which the various valves are affected by chronic rheumatic heart disease?

3   What are the main causes of mitral stenosis?

Answers

1   **Acute rheumatic fever and chronic rheumatic heart disease**

After an attack of acute rheumatic fever the heart returns to normal in approximately 50% of cases. In the other 50% the condition rumbles on occultly causing symptomatic disease after an interval that is typically 15–20 years in the West, although it may be as short as 4–5 years or as long as 30–40 years. A short interval is particularly likely in developing countries where chronic rheumatic heart disease is often seen in children.

2   **The approximate frequencies with which the various valves are affected by chronic rheumatic heart disease**

● Mitral valve: 80%
● Aortic valve: 50%
● Aortic and mitral valves together: 20%
● Tricuspid valve: 10%
● Pulmonary valve: 1%

3   **Causes of mitral stenosis**

Chronic rheumatic heart disease is by far the commonest cause of mitral stenosis. Very occasionally it may be congenital. Obstruction of the mitral valve may also be caused by an atrial myxoma.

Rheumatic mitral stenosis (i): pathology; circulatory effects

Questions

4   What percentage of patients with mitral stenosis are aware

of past acute rheumatic fever? What percentage of patients are female?

5i   What is the average cross-sectional area of the normal mitral valve? What is it likely to be in tight mitral stenosis? What are the main haemodynamic effects of mitral stenosis upon the systemic circulation?

ii   Describe the changes that occur with mitral stenosis in the valve, the heart, and the lungs. What is the effect of the development of pulmonary hypertension?

Answers

4   Mitral stenosis and previous rheumatic fever

Only about 50% of patients with rheumatic mitral stenosis are aware of having had acute rheumatic fever. About two-thirds of the patients with mitral stenosis are female.

5   Effects of mitral stenosis

i   Normally the cross-sectional area of the mitral valve is 4-5 cm^2. In tight mitral stenosis this may be reduced to < 1 cm^2. Systemically, obstruction of the mitral valve leads to a small stroke volume and a low cardiac output.

ii   In the *valve*, fusion of the commissures occurs, together with thickening of the valve cusps, and thickening and shortening of the chordae tendineae. Eventually calcification of the valve cusps or ring may occur. Initially the main change in the *heart* is enlargement of the left atrium due to obstruction of the mitral valve which in a sense often 'protects' the left ventricle. As it enlarges the atrium may become electrically unstable, resulting in atrial fibrillation. Due to stasis, thrombus may form in the enlarged left atrium, particularly with atrial fibrillation.

In the *lungs*, because it leads to damning back of the blood, pulmonary congestion occurs. In response to the congestion, with time the walls of the pulmonary capillaries thicken. Both the congestion and thickening of the walls of the pulmonary capillaries render the lungs stiff and less than normally compliant, increase the work of breathing and contribute to the breathlessness associated with the condition. When the pressure in the left atrium and pulmonary capillaries reaches about 25 mmHg frank pulmonary oedema may occur, although the thickening of the capillaries tends to protect against this.

In about 20% of cases the increased pressure within the pulmonary vasculature causes reflex vasoconstriction of the pulmonary arteries. Initially this results in reduction of the flow of blood through the lungs, partially relieving the pulmonary congestion. For a while the patient may appear better and less breathless than before, but eventually the vasoconstriction of the pulmonary arteries results in pulmonary hypertension with pressures in the pulmonary artery up to two to three times normal, leading to dilatation and hypertrophy of the right ventricle, functional tricuspid regurgitation due to dilatation of the valvular ring, and right ventricular failure.

Rheumatic mitral stenosis (ii): symptoms, signs, investigation, treatment

Questions

6   What are (i) the symptoms, and (ii) the signs of mitral stenosis?

7   What are the main ECG and chest x-ray changes associated with mitral stenosis? What are the modern specific investigations of the condition?

8   Describe the medical treatment of mitral stenosis. What are the main indications for surgical intervention?

Answers

6   The symptoms and signs of mitral stenosis

i   *Symptoms.* These follow from what has been said above and are breathlessness due mainly to stiffness of the lungs, and reduced exercise tolerance due to breathlessness and low cardiac output. Orthopnoea and attacks of frank pulmonary oedema may occur. Congestion of the lungs may lead to winter bronchitis and haemoptysis. Particularly in patients who are in atrial fibrillation, emboli may arise from either atrium causing pulmonary infarction, or ischaemia or infarction of brain, gut, kidney, a limb, or occasionally even occlusion of a coronary artery. Eventually oedema of the legs may occur.

ii   *Signs.* Generally, the prolonged low cardiac output often leads to weight loss and cyanosis with a particular manifestation on the cheeks known as a *malar flush*. The pulse is usually small, and may be fibrillating.

●   *In the heart*, to a large extent the signs depend upon the mobility of the valve. The high pressure generated in the large left atrium holds the valve open until ventricular systole is under way. If the valve is mobile a very high velocity closure is then effected producing a *loud first sound* that can be felt as a *tapping apex*. Similarly if the valve is mobile its sudden opening under high atrial pressure produces an *opening snap just after the second heart sound*, best heard to the left of the lower sternum. If the valve is calcified and immobile the situation may well be the complete opposite of that just described, in that the first sound is soft, and the opening snap absent.

The rumbling character of the murmur as blood passes through the stenosed valve is described on page 22. It is best heard at the apex, using the bell of the stethoscope applied very lightly to the skin with the patient lying over to the left to bring the apex closer. With sinus rhythm the murmur becomes louder towards its end as the atrium contracts and pushes extra blood through. This is the presystolic crescendo, and does not occur with atrial fibrillation because with that condition there is no co-ordinated atrial contraction.

● As pulmonary hypertension develops the right ventricle becomes palpable and signs of tricuspid regurgitation and right ventricular failure occur.

7   Specific investigations

● *The ECG* may show either sinus rhythm or atrial fibrillation. In patients in sinus rhythm the P wave may be large and bifid due to electrical conduction in the large left atrium taking longer than in the right atrium.

● *Chest x-ray.* The commonest abnormality is enlargement of the left atrium which is seen as a double outline on the right side of the cardiac shadow and as enlargement of the left border of the heart just below the pulmonary artery. Calcification of the valve may be seen to the left of the vertebral column. The lungs may appear congested and Kerley B lines and frank pulmonary oedema may be visible. A description of these changes is given on page 38. With the development of pulmonary hypertension the proximal pulmonary arteries are often dilated, and blood may be diverted to the upper lobes causing a decrease in prominence of the vessels to the lower lobes.

● *Specifically* mitral stenosis is assessed by various echocardiographic techniques, making cardiac catheterisation

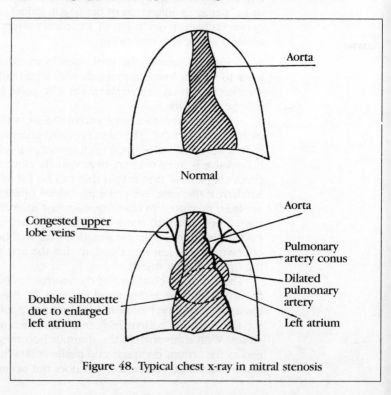

Figure 48. Typical chest x-ray in mitral stenosis

usually unnecessary. With these techniques delayed closure of the mitral valve, thickening of the valve cusps and enlargement of the left atrium may be observed.

8 Medical treatment and indications for surgery

Apart from prophylactic antibiotics before dentistry or other instrumentation (see page 210), symptomless minor mitral stenosis does not require specific treatment. The onset of atrial fibrillation should be treated with digitalis as described on page 45, and with anticoagulants as described on page 67. Oedema should be treated with diuretics, and chest infection with a broad spectrum antibiotic.

The indications for surgery are often a matter of fine judgement, and are firstly onset of symptoms such as exercise limitation or pulmonary oedema, and secondly systemic emboli despite adequate anticoagulation.

Mitral regurgitation (i): classification; haemodynamic effects

Questions

9   List the causes of mitral regurgitation, classifying them according to anatomical site and writing a line or two about the underlying pathology of each.

10   What are the haemodynamic effects of well developed mitral regurgitation upon the stroke volume, the character of the pulse, the left ventricle and the lungs?

Answers

9   Causes of mitral regurgitation

These are best classified anatomically as follows:

● *Valve cusps*

a   *Chronic rheumatic heart disease* due to scarring, retraction and distortion of the valve cusps, the valve ring and chordae tendineae.

b   *Mitral valve prolapse (floppy valve syndrome)* due to mucinous or myxoedematous change within the valve, and an associated increase in the area of the cusp and sometimes elongation of the chordae tendineae. As a consequence the cusp goes up into the left atrium during systole. A similar condition may occur with Marfan's, the Ehlers–Danlos and straight back syndromes.

c   *Infective endocarditis* due to the infective process destroying the valve or chordae tendineae.

● *Papillary muscle*

a   *Dysfunction* due to ischaemia or cardiomyopathy.

b   *Rupture* due to acute myocardial infarction.

● *Chordae tendineae*

a   *Elongation* as part of the mitral valve prolapse syndrome.

b   *Shortening* due to chronic rheumatic heart disease.

c   *Rupture* due to infective endocarditis, or sudden stretching of the left ventricle as a result of left ventricular failure due to myocardial infarction.

● *Valve ring. Dilatation*, as part of the dilatation of the left ventricle that may occur with severe left ventricular failure. This type of mitral regurgitation may resolve with treatment of the underlying heart failure.

10   Haemodynamic effects

Because the left atrium is very compliant and the pressure within it is low, well developed mitral regurgitation is associated with the rapid regurgitation of a large volume of blood into the left atrium during ventricular systole. As a result of the large volume of blood that flows backwards and forwards between the atrium and ventricle the stroke volume may be two or three times normal, much of the blood being ejected rapidly into the left atrium before the aortic valve has opened. In the systemic circulation the *rapid* ejection of much of the stroke volume into the left atrium results in a small volume pulse of a *rapid* or *jerky* character.

Despite the ease and completeness with which the ventricle empties and the sinus tachycardia that often accompanies it, mitral regurgitation of any severity usually leads to dilatation of the left ventricle, although if the condition is of acute onset, due for instance to rupture of a papillary muscle following myocardial infarction, initially the heart size may be normal.

In the *lungs* congestion may occur, particularly with the onset of left ventricular failure.

Mitral regurgitation (ii): symptoms, signs, investigation, treatment
Questions

11i   Describe the symptoms and the signs of mitral regurgitation.
   ii   List the complications that occur occasionally with mitral valve prolapse.
12   Describe the main chest x-ray changes associated with mitral regurgitation. How else may the condition be investigated?
13   How is mitral regurgitation treated? What are the indications for surgical intervention?

Answers

11   The symptoms and signs of mitral regurgitation; complications of mitral valve prolapse

i   The *symptoms* of mitral regurgitation vary with the cause and severity of the condition. Mitral valve prolapse is usually an incidental symptomless finding. Rheumatic mitral regurgitation usually presents with increasing breathlessness years after an attack of rheumatic fever. On the other hand rupture of a papillary muscle following myocardial infarction or rupture of a valve cusp due to infective endocarditis may well present with severe sudden breathlessness due to acute pulmonary oedema and with shock due to low cardiac output.

The *signs* of mitral regurgitation also vary with the cause and severity of the condition. Prolapse of the mitral valve is typically associated with a click in the middle of systole and a short late systolic murmur. Conditions in which dysfunction of a papillary muscle or chordae is only partial tend to be associated with regurgitation late in systole and the production of a late systolic murmur. On the other hand the shrunken distorted valve of chronic rheumatic mitral regurgitation, or a valve that is ruptured, tends to be incompetent throughout the whole of systole and to produce a pan-systolic murmur. Classically but not always this murmur is loudest at the apex and radiates to the axilla. If it is loud enough, it may produce a thrill.

Other signs of severe mitral regurgitation are a small jerky pulse, enlargement of the left ventricle with a displaced sustained apex beat, and a third heart sound. Any parasternal heave is likely to be due to the large expansile left atrium associated with the condition or to dilatation of the left ventricle, rather than right ventricular hypertrophy.

ii   *Mitral valve prolapse* is usually symptomless, but very occasionally is associated with chest pain, ventricular ectopic beats and arrhythmias, and ulceration of the valve cusps predisposing to thrombus formation, arterial emboli and infective endocarditis.

12   Investigations

•   *Chest x-ray*. The typical change associated with mitral regurgitation is selective enlargement of the left atrium. In severe disease of any standing the cardiac shadow is enlarged. With mitral regurgitation of rheumatic origin calcification may be seen in the valve.

•   *With modern Doppler and echocardiography*, cardiac catheterisation is usually required only to confirm or exclude coexisting coronary artery disease.

13   Treatment

Apart from prophylactic antibiotics before dentistry or other instrumentation (see page 210), symptomless mitral regurgitation does not require specific treatment. Left ventricular failure is treated along the lines discussed on page 43. Surgery with either repair or replacement of the valve is indicated for severe chronic mitral regurgitation causing significant symptoms despite medical treatment, or for severe regurgitation of sudden onset due to rupture of a valve cusp, chordae or papillary muscle.

Aortic stenosis (i): classification; circulatory effects
Questions

Question 14 is about aortic stenosis in general, and questions 15-18 about valvular aortic stenosis in particular.

14 List the causes of aortic stenosis, classifying them according to anatomical site.

15 What are the main effects of aortic stenosis on the heart and systemic circulation? What is the pressure gradient across the valve likely to be in severe aortic stenosis?

Answers

14 Causes of aortic stenosis

Aortic stenosis is classified as supravalvular, valvular and subvalvular as follows:

● *Supravalvular*. A very rare cause of aortic stenosis that may be familial and is due to a fibrous ring or hypoplasia of the aorta.

● *Valvular*. The commonest cause of aortic stenosis, it may be subdivided into:

a *Calcification of a congenitally bicuspid valve*. This occurs in later life and overall is the commonest cause of aortic stenosis.

b *Chronic rheumatic valvular disease*.

c *Calcification in old age of a tricuspid valve*.

● *Subvalvular*. A rare condition due either to a fibrous ring or to hypertrophic cardiomyopathy (HOCM).

15 The main effects of aortic stenosis upon the heart and systemic circulation

The heart responds to the obstruction caused by aortic stenosis by increasing its work and power of contraction, that is by increasing systolic tension. Like any muscle required to work against an increased load the heart muscle responds by hypertrophy. Only late in the disease does dilatation occur. In the systemic circulation the obstruction of the valve is associated with a small stroke volume, a small slow rising pulse, low blood pressure and low cardiac output. In severe aortic stenosis the pressure difference during systole between the left ventricle and aorta is often greater than 50-60 mmHg.

Aortic stenosis (ii): symptoms, signs, investigation, treatment
Questions

16i What is the triad of symptoms associated with aortic stenosis?

ii What are the signs of aortic stenosis?

17 How is aortic stenosis investigated?

18 How is it treated?

Answers

16   Symptoms and signs of aortic stenosis

Aortic stenosis may be symptomless. In symptomatic cases a triad of symptoms is recognised:
- *Angina of effort* due to low cardiac output and any coexisting coronary artery disease.
- *Breathlessness* on exertion or at night due to left ventricular failure.
- *Syncope or dizziness*, especially during or just after exertion, due to low cardiac output.

Signs

Due to obstruction of the aortic valve, systole takes longer than normal. The result is a slow rising pulse of small volume, the character of which is often most easily appreciated in the carotid artery. Because of obstruction, the blood pressure is low with a small pulse pressure.

Aortic stenosis may affect the function of both atria. On the right side, an a wave may be visible in the jugular venous pulse. This is due to the hypertrophied left ventricle bulging into the right ventricle and interfering with right ventricular filling. As a consequence the right atrium contracts against increased resistance and as explained on page 16 produces the observed a wave. On the left side, as it pushes blood into the thickened stiff left ventricle the left atrium may hypertrophy and dilate producing a palpable beat which as described on page 17 may be felt as a second or double apex.

The left ventricular apex itself is *sustained*. A *thrill* may be palpable over the aortic area at the base of the heart. Because the valve is immobile and does not close completely, the aortic component of the *second heart sound is usually reduced or absent*. As the atrium contracts at the end of systole and squeezes a last drop of blood into the already partially filled thickened left ventricle, the ventricle may creak producing *a fourth heart sound* in response to the atrial contraction. *The characteristic harsh systolic murmur* is maximal over the aortic area and radiates along the carotid arteries into the neck. Often a non-significant short diastolic murmur is audible along the left sternal edge due to minimal regurgitation resulting from failure of the valve cusps to close completely.

17   Investigations

- *Chest x-ray*. Usually the heart size is normal or a little enlarged. Calcification of the valve is best seen on lateral chest x-ray or with cardiac screening.
- *ECG* characteristically shows the changes of left ventricular hypertrophy described on page 39. If calcification of the valve involves the conducting tissue, heart block or bundle branch block may be evident.

●   *Echocardiography*. This investigation gives information about the pathology of the valve, the thickness of the left ventricular wall and the size of the left ventricular cavity. Doppler echocardiography gives information about the gradient across the valve.

●   *Cardiac catheterisation* allows direct assessment of the severity of the disease by measurement of the systolic pressure gradient across the valve, the end diastolic pressure and the size of the left ventricular cavity. At the same time the state of the coronary arteries may be assessed by coronary arteriography.

18   Treatment

Apart from prophylactic antibiotics before dentistry and other instrumentation, symptomless aortic stenosis does not require specific treatment. Since the primary abnormality is a mechanical obstruction the treatment of symptomatic aortic stenosis is surgical replacement of the valve, together with coronary artery bypass surgery if indicated. Any heart failure should be treated medically before surgery.

Aortic regurgitation (i): classification and circulatory effects

Questions

19   List the causes of aortic regurgitation.
20   What are the main effects of aortic regurgitation upon the heart and systemic circulation?

Answers

19   Causes of aortic regurgitation

●   *Distortion of a valve cusp*, due for instance to chronic rheumatic heart disease, or less commonly a collagenosis such as rheumatoid arthritis.

●   *Perforation of a valve cusp* due to infective endocarditis.

●   *Dilatation of the aortic ring* due to severe hypertension, dissecting aneurysm, tertiary syphilis, Reiter's disease, ankylosing spondylitis and Marfan's syndrome.

●   *Prolapse of the valve into a ventricular septal defect (VSD)*. This occurs in about 15% of VSDs.

20   The main effects of aortic regurgitation upon the heart and systemic circulation

The effects of aortic regurgitation upon the heart and systemic circulation follow from the ejection of a large volume of blood into the aorta and regurgitation of part of it back into the heart. The movement of such a large volume of blood into the peripheral circulation and then back into the heart produces a large volume pulse. The diastolic pressure associated with the condition is usually low due to peripheral dilatation and the movement of blood back into the heart from the systemic circulation. The increased volume of blood in the heart at the end of diastole leads to an increase of end diastolic pressure that gradually causes the heart to dilate and the stroke volume to increase by two, three or even four times normal.

Aortic regurgitation (ii): symptoms, signs, investigation, treatment

Questions

21 What are the main symptoms and the main signs of aortic regurgitation? What is Corrigan's sign, Quincke's sign and the Austin Flint murmur?
22 How is aortic regurgitation investigated?
23 How is it treated?

Answers

21 The symptoms and signs of aortic regurgitation

In many cases, aortic regurgitation is an incidental finding in a symptomless patient. The commonest presenting symptom is *breathlessness*, initially on exertion, due to developing left ventricular failure. *Angina of effort* may also occur due either to poor perfusion of the coronary arteries as a result of the low diastolic pressure that occurs with the condition, or more rarely to syphylitic aortitis involving a coronary ostium.

Signs

Following on from what has been said, the pulse is bounding or like a waterhammer (named after a Victorian toy called a waterhammer because of the thud produced within the toy as water under vacuum moved suddenly from one end of a tube to the other). The best way of eliciting this sign is described on page 12. When the bounding nature of the pulse is visible in the carotid arteries in the neck the pulse is referred to as *Corrigan's sign*; when visible in the nails it is referred to as *Quincke's sign*.

In severe disease the apex beat is sustained and displaced laterally. On auscultation several murmurs may be heard. The typical decrescendo diastolic murmur that sounds like the twanging of a pair of cymbals is usually heard best along the left sternal edge with the patient sitting up, leaning slightly forward and holding their breath. In addition an ejection systolic murmur may be heard at the base of the heart. In the presence of gross aortic regurgitation this is due to the greatly increased stroke volume rushing through the aorta, and not to aortic stenosis. At the apex a third murmur may be audible. This is a diastolic rumble similar to the murmur of mitral stenosis from which it is distinguished by the absence of an opening snap (and by echocardiography). It is due to fluttering of the anterior cusp of the mitral valve as blood flows back past it into the heart in diastole, and is known as the *Austin Flint murmur*.

22 Investigations

● Except where the aetiology of the condition is clearly known, *serology for syphilis* should be checked in all cases of aortic regurgitation. In disease of any severity the ECG will show the changes of left ventricular hypertrophy (see page 39), and chest x-ray cardiac enlargement and dilatation of the aortic root.

● *Echocardiography* will show the size of the left ventricular cavity, the aortic root and give information about the regurgitant jet.

● *Cardiac catheterisation* may be performed prior to operation, or for cases in which more information is required.

23 Treatment

Apart from prophylactic antibiotics when indicated, with the exception of the reservation discussed below, symptomless aortic regurgitation does not require specific treatment, although young patients should be advised to avoid excessive exercise as it may cause the cavity of the left ventricle to dilate. In those with symptoms, surgical replacement of the valve is indicated.

Patients who are asymptomatic should be seen at regular intervals so that if necessary surgery may be advised if irreversible left ventricular damage seems likely to develop. The accepted way of monitoring these patients is to review them regularly, looking for any increase of heart size on clinical examination, chest x-ray, echocardiogram or electrocardiogram. The function of the heart may also be assessed by formal exercise testing.

Further Reading

Braunwald E (ed) (1984). *Heart Disease*, 2nd edition. WB
        Saunders, Philadelphia. Chapter 31, valvular heart disease.
Weatherall DJ, Ledingham JGG, Warrell DA (eds) (1987). *Oxford
        Textbook of Medicine*, 2nd edition. Oxford University Press,
        Oxford. Valve disease, pp 13.281-304.

Chapter 12
Congenital Heart Disease

Atrial septal defect (ASD); ventricular septal defect (VSD); Eisenmenger's syndrome

Questions

1i Briefly describe the nature of the lesion in the ostium secundum type of ASD. What are its main effects upon the circulation and the heart? What is the natural history of the condition? What are its main symptoms and signs? What complications are likely? How is it treated?

ii What is an ostium primum ASD? In what important respects does it differ from the ostium secundum lesion? How is it treated?

2 Do VSDs close spontaneously? Upon what do the symptoms and signs produced by a VSD depend? What are the main symptoms and signs of a small VSD and a large VSD? What are the main complications of a large VSD? How are VSDs treated?

3i What is Eisenmenger's syndrome? What are the main symptoms and signs of the condition? Why is it difficult to treat?

ii Which of the commoner congenital heart conditions is or may be associated with a right to left shunt?

Answers

1   Atrial septal defect

i *Ostium secundum ASD* is due to failure of development of the septum secundum. As a consequence there is shunting of blood from left to right at atrial level. Depending upon the size of the defect the flow across the heart may be three or four times as much as through the systemic circulation. The main effect upon the heart is to cause enlargement of the right atrium, the right ventricle and the pulmonary artery and veins; the left ventricle and aorta are small. Pulmonary hypertension occurs in about 10% of cases, adding to any right sided heart failure.

• *Natural history, symptoms and signs.* Patients with ostium secundum ASD often do not develop symptoms until they are aged 40-50 when breathlessness occurs due to heart failure, particularly with the onset of atrial fibrillation. *The signs* of an ostium secundum ASD are often subtle and easily missed. Due to the increased flow of blood through the right side of the heart, the right ventricle may be abnormally palpable and a systolic flow murmur may be audible over the pulmonary artery in the second left intercostal space. Because of the increased stroke volume on the right side of the heart, right ventricular systole is prolonged causing delayed closure of the pulmonary valve and wide splitting of the second heart sound heard best over the pulmonary area. With large ASDs the increased flow of blood through the tricuspid valve as right ventricular filling occurs may produce a soft diastolic murmur along the left sternal edge.

● *Complications and treatment*. Most patients with ASD eventually develop heart failure. About 10% develop pulmonary hypertension. To forestall these occurrences, ASDs should be closed surgically, exceptions being patients with Eisenmenger's syndrome and patients aged over about 65 years.

ii *Ostium primum ASD* is uncommon, occurring in about 5–10% of ASDs. It is caused by failure of the septum primum to develop normally and is associated with abnormalities of the adjacent atrioventricular valvular apparatus. As a result in 75% of cases the anterior cusp of the mitral valve is cleft causing mitral regurgitation. Often this is associated with an increase of the shunt, blood flowing from the left ventricle to the right atrium through the apex of the cleft, as well as from the left atrium. Because of its proximity to the A-V node and bundle of His the condition is prone to heart block and other abnormalities of conduction.

● The signs of the condition are a compound of the signs of an ostium secundum ASD and of mitral regurgitation. Because of the mitral regurgitation, conduction defects and a tendency to early development of pulmonary hypertension, ostium primum lesions have more severe effects than ostium secundum lesions, and usually present in childhood or early adulthood. Except when the shunt is small, the defect should be closed and the mitral valve repaired surgically.

2 Ventricular septal defect

● Defects between the left and right ventricles occur at several sites in the septal wall. Those near the aortic valve may be associated with prolapse of the valve and aortic regurgitation, and do not close spontaneously. Those beneath the septal cusp of the tricuspid valve tend to close spontaneously or to become smaller. This is most likely during childhood, but may occur at any age. Other VSDs are associated with congenital conditions such as Fallot's tetralogy.

● *Symptoms and signs* produced by a VSD depend upon its size and location. Typically the sound produced by a VSD is a pan-systolic murmur loudest to the left of the sternum over the third or fourth intercostal space. A small defect producing no symptoms or important haemodynamic effects may produce a murmur and thrill out of proportion to its clinical significance—*maladie de Roger*. Large VSDs are seen mainly in children and are rare in adults. A large VSD may be associated with a shunt that is three or four times the systemic output. The result of a large shunt is an increase in the work of both the left and the right sides of the heart. The main physical signs of a large VSD are therefore a sustained hyperdynamic apex beat, an abnormally palpable right ventricle, and a pan-systolic murmur. If the increased flow of blood back from the lungs through the mitral valve is sufficiently great a functional diastolic mitral murmur may also be heard at the apex. When a VSD is associated with aortic regurgitation the murmurs produced are audible in both systole and diastole.

• *Complications and treatment*. VSDs of any size may be affected by infective endocarditis. Large VSDs may cause heart failure and be associated with the development of pulmonary hypertension. With the exception of prophylactic antibiotics, small symptomless VSDs do not require treatment. Large ones that are producing symptoms should be closed surgically before pulmonary hypertension develops.

3   Eisenmenger's syndrome

i   Usually openings between the two sides of the circulation are associated with shunting of blood from the high pressure left side to the low pressure right side. Eisenmenger's syndrome is reversal of the shunt due to the development of severe pulmonary hypertension and the development of greater pressures on the right side of the heart than on the left. This results in venous blood entering the left side of the heart, causing cyanosis. Eisenmenger's syndrome may develop with a VSD, an ASD or persistent ductus.

• *Symptoms and signs*. The main symptom of the condition is increasing breathlessness. Grossly, the main signs are cyanosis and clubbing. In the cardiovascular system the symptoms and signs are those of pulmonary hypertension. The age of onset of the condition depends upon the underlying cause. Usually it is early life, but in the case of an ostium secundum ASD middle age may have occurred before any pulmonary hypertension is severe enough to reverse the shunt.

• *Treatment*. There is no specific treatment for the condition. Any attempt to close the defect and establish a normal circulation through the pulmonary arteries merely makes the pulmonary hypertension worse and leads to circulatory failure.

ii   The commonest congenital conditions associated with right to left shunt and cyanosis are those listed above causing Eisenmenger's syndrome, and Fallot's tetralogy.

Fallot's tetralogy; persistent ductus arteriosus; coarctation of the aorta; Ebstein's anomaly and dextrocardia

Questions

4   Describe the essentials of Fallot's tetralogy. What is the main symptom associated with it? What is the explanation of the squatting position often adopted by the patient? How is the condition treated?

5   What is a persistent ductus arteriosus? What are the main physical signs associated with it? What complications is it subject to? How is it treated?

6   What is coarctation of the aorta? With what other conditions
may it be associated? What are the main complications to which it
is subject? What are the main physical signs? How is it treated?
7   What is Ebstein's anomaly?
8   What abnormality of the intestines is often associated with
dextrocardia?
9   What is Lutembacher's syndrome?

Answers

4   Fallot's tetralogy

This is a congenital cyanotic condition of the heart consisting of a
large VSD, infundibular or occasionally valvular pulmonary stenosis,
an overriding aorta, that is an aorta overriding and taking blood
from both the left and right ventricles, and right ventricular
hypertrophy. The main symptom of the condition is breathlessness.
The characteristic squatting position adopted by patients with
Fallot's increases peripheral resistance and pressure within the
aorta, thereby tending to block the flow of venous blood into the
aorta from the right ventricle. As a consequence the oxygen
content of the arterial blood is increased. Treatment is by surgical
correction of the pulmonary stenosis and repair of the VSD.

5   Persistent ductus arteriosus

●   Normally the ductus connecting the pulmonary artery to the
aorta closes shortly after birth. Its persistence is associated with a
left to right shunt.
●   The main physical signs of a persistent ductus are a
collapsing pulse with a low diastolic pressure as blood flows from
the aorta to the low pressure pulmonary circulation. The left
ventricle is enlarged. Due to the continuous flow of blood through
the lesion in both systole and diastole, a machinery murmur with
systolic and diastolic components, and possibly a thrill, is audible
and heard best in the second left intercostal space.
●   *The main complications* of the condition are heart failure
due to increased cardiac output; pulmonary hypertension in a
proportion of patients; and the risk of infective endocarditis.
●   *Treatment* is by surgical closure, except in patients who have
already developed pulmonary hypertension.

6   Coarctation of the aorta

This is a narrowing of the aorta, in the adult usually just below the
origin of the left subclavian artery. As a consequence relative
ischaemia occurs in the lower half of the body, although the
obstruction is partially bypassed and blood carried to the distal
aorta by a mesh of collateral vessels in the thorax. The condition is
commoner in males than females by a ratio of $4:1$, and may be
associated with a number of congenital abnormalities such as
bicuspid aortic valve, Turner's syndrome, persistent ductus, septal
defects and mitral regurgitation. It may lead to hypertension in the

upper half of the body. The cause of the hypertension is unknown, but may be due to the increased systolic tension developed by the left ventricle in response to the obstruction, or to activation of the angiotensin-renin system in the ischaemic lower half of the body, or both. Apart from hypertension, the other complications of the condition are heart failure that may be associated with normal blood pressure or hypertension, subarachnoid haemorrhage and infective endocarditis.

● *The main physical signs* of the condition are absence, or reduction and delay of the femoral pulse compared to the radial pulse, and visible collateral blood vessels on the back over which a flow hum may be heard.

● *Treatment* is by surgical excision of the defect, or grafting if the defect is long.

7 Ebstein's anomaly

This is a congenital defect in which the origin of the tricuspid valve is beneath the true atrioventricular ring resulting in a small right ventricle. In addition the anterior cusp of the tricuspid valve is voluminous and prolapses into the right atrium producing varying degrees of tricuspid incompetence. In 80% of cases there is an associated ASD with a right to left shunt producing cyanosis.

8 Dextrocardia

This may occur alone or with transposition of the abdominal viscera. Apart from the fact that it may confuse the attending doctors, it is not clinically important.

9 Lutembacher's syndrome

This is the rare association of a congenital ostium secundum atrial septal defect and mitral stenosis that is usually acquired but may be congenital.

Further Reading

Braunwald E (ed) (1984). *Heart Disease*, 2nd edition. WB
    Saunders, Philadelphia. Chapters 28, congenital heart disease
    in infancy and childhood; 29, congenital heart disease in the
    adult.
Weatherall DJ, Ledingham JGG, Warrell DA (eds) (1987). *Oxford
    Textbook of Medicine*, 2nd edition. Oxford University Press,
    Oxford. Congenital heart disease, pp 13.23-77.

Chapter 13 Pulmonary Hypertension

Pathophysiology
Questions

1 What are the ranges of the normal pulmonary artery systolic and diastolic pressures?

2 What is the common response in the pulmonary arteries that leads to the production of pulmonary hypertension? What are the conditions or groups of conditions with which this common response is associated?

3 What are the main effects of pulmonary hypertension upon the main proximal pulmonary arteries, the heart and systemic circulation?

Answers

1   Normal pulmonary artery pressures

The pulmonary circulation is a low pressure system within which the normal systolic pressure is 15–30 mmHg, and the normal diastolic pressure is 5–15 mmHg.

2   Mechanism of pulmonary hypertension

With the exception of primary pulmonary hypertension, which is a very rare condition, pulmonary hypertension is invariably a common response of the pulmonary arteries to disease of several kinds. The initial event is constriction of the smaller branches of the pulmonary arteries. With time the smooth muscle in the arterial wall hypertrophies and the condition becomes irreversible. The conditions which may result in spasm of the pulmonary vasculature and pulmonary hypertension are:

● *Alveolar hypoxia*, due for instance to severe chronic obstructive airways disease.

● *Pulmonary venous hypertension* due to mitral stenosis.

● *Pulmonary vascular distension* caused by a high flow of blood through the pulmonary arteries with large left to right shunts.

● *Obliteration of the pulmonary microvasculature* by recurrent small pulmonary emboli.

3   Effect upon the heart and circulation

The main proximal pulmonary arteries dilate, begin to resemble the aorta, and may develop atheroma. Because of dilatation of the main pulmonary artery the pulmonary valve cusps may become incompetent. In the heart hypertrophy of the right atrium and right ventricle occurs, often with dilatation of the atrioventricular ring. In the systemic circulation, the obstruction of the pulmonary circulation results in a low cardiac output and a small pulse volume. As the pressure in the pulmonary system comes to equal the pressure within the systemic circulation any shunt that is present is reversed.

Symptoms, signs, chest x-ray, treatment
Questions

4   What are (i) the symptoms, and (ii) the signs of pulmonary hypertension? What is the Graham Steell murmur?
5   What are the chest x-ray changes associated with pulmonary hypertension?
6   How is the condition treated?

Answers

4   Symptoms and signs

i   Initially the symptoms and signs are those of the causative disease, but as pulmonary hypertension develops and becomes severe it comes to dominate the clinical picture causing breathlessness at rest, sometimes anginal-like chest pain due to the load on the right ventricle, and also effort syncope due to low cardiac output.

ii   *Signs* of the condition are a loud pulmonary component of the second heart sound due to high pressure in the pulmonary circulation causing high velocity closure of the pulmonary valve; a parasternal heave due to right ventricular hypertrophy; and a large a wave in the jugular venous pulse due, as described on page 16, to the right atrium contracting against the increased resistance to filling of the hypertrophied stiff, non-compliant right ventricle. Incompetence of the pulmonary valve cusps is associated with a decrescendo diastolic murmur along the sternal edge resembling the murmur of aortic regurgitation from which it is distinguished by a small pulse volume and absence of a hyperdynamic peripheral circulation. When pulmonary regurgitation is associated with pulmonary hypertension due to mitral stenosis the pulmonary diastolic murmur is known as the *Graham Steell murmur*. Dilatation of the atrioventricular ring on the right side of the heart results in tricuspid regurgitation and its associated murmur and a large wave in the jugular venous pulse that for historical reasons is known as a v wave although it occurs at the time of the c wave. In addition if the foramen ovale has remained unsealed throughout the patient's life, the high pressure in the right atrium will open it and blood will shunt from right to left.

5 Chest x-ray

The heart is usually of a normal size until right ventricular failure occurs. The dilated main pulmonary artery may be seen as a bulge to the left of the mediastinum, between the aorta and the left border of the heart. The main branches of the left and right pulmonary arteries are also enlarged in their proximal parts, only to be pruned in the periphery by the severe vasoconstriction that initiates the condition and results in abnormally translucent peripheral lung fields.

6 Treatment

Mitral stenosis should be relieved surgically before pulmonary hypertension develops. By the time the pressure in the pulmonary circulation has risen to any degree it is too late to close any shunt. In case it is due to occult pulmonary emboli, anticoagulants are often given in cases in which the cause of pulmonary hypertension is obscure. Rest and diuretics are prescribed for right heart failure.

Further Reading

Weatherall DJ, Ledingham JGG, Warrell DA (eds) (1987). *Oxford Textbook of Medicine*, 2nd edition. Oxford University Press, Oxford. Pulmonary hypertension, pp 13.342-50.

Case I **An Ill Lady:
Miss U-R, aged
51 years**

An unmarried clerk living with her elderly mother in a corporation house.

History of present condition

Admitted to hospital with a 2 month history of a 'flu-like illness associated with generalised weakness, aching of the muscles, feelings of being hot then cold, poor appetite and 12 lb weight loss. Because of the loss of appetite her family doctor had a barium meal performed which showed a small sliding hiatus hernia with reflux.

During the week prior to admission she had developed breathlessness and swelling of the ankles that responded to frusemide 40 mg daily.

Past medical history

Two years previously prolapse of the mitral valve had been confirmed by echocardiography after an apical systolic murmur had been discovered during investigaion of blackouts that were subsequently shown to be due to grand mal epilepsy. No further blackouts had occurred since starting treatment with phenytoin.

Relevant direct questions

Drugs: phenytoin 100 mg three times per day; frusemide 40 mg daily.

Examination

Pale unwell looking pyrexial middle-aged lady with a suggestion of clubbing of the finger nails. Temperature 38°C.

Cardiovasculature system (CVS)

Pulse 90 regular, good volume.
BP 120/80 lying and standing.
Jugular venous pulse (JVP) not visible.

On palpation

Apex: sustained and displaced to the anterior axillary line in the fifth intercostal space.
Right ventricle impalpable.

On auscultation

A loud pan-systolic murmur audible at the apex, radiating towards the axilla.

Respiratory system (RS)

At the lung bases a few late inspiratory crackles were audible.

Abdominal system (AS)

The only abnormality was a palpable spleen, about 3 cm below the left costal margin.

Initial observations and investigations

On the ward Miss U-R continued to be unwell and pyrexial, temperature 37.5–38.5°C. Initial investigations gave the following results:
Haemoglobin (Hb): 10.3 g% with normal indices and a normochromic blood film.
White blood cells (WBC): 5500 with a normal differential.
Erythrocyte sedimentation rate (ESR): 80 mm/hour.
Biochemical screen and ECG normal.
Chest x-ray: slight cardiomegaly.

Miss U-R

Questions

1   What diagnosis is suggested by the history, physical findings and initial investigations?
2   What specific further investigations would you have ordered?

Answers

1   The diagnosis of Miss U-R's case

The history of general unwellness for several weeks, the development of symptoms suggestive of cardiac failure, the past history of an abnormal heart valve and the findings on examination of persistent pyrexia, a hint of finger clubbing, an enlarged heart, a loud systolic murmur and a palpable spleen, and the findings on investigation of a normochromic anaemia and a high ESR all suggest that until proved otherwise Miss U-R was suffering from infective endocarditis.

2   The specific further investigation of Miss U-R's case

The specific investigations in a case of suspected infective endocarditis are (a) serial blood cultures, and (b) echocardiography of the heart valves. In Miss U-R's case each of four blood cultures yielded a pure growth of *Streptococcus viridans* sensitive to penicillin. Echocardiography showed vegetations on the posterior cusp and the chordae tendineae of the anterior cusp of the mitral valve.

Further history about Miss U-R

Because infective endocarditis was so strongly suspected, whilst the results of blood culture were awaited, treatment was begun with boluses of intravenous benzylpenicillin 1.2 g (2 mega units) every 4 hours and gentamicin 80 mg every 8 hours. Despite this Miss U-R's temperature failed to settle, and after 2½ weeks she was transferred to a cardiac unit where the mitral valve was replaced with an artificial prosthesis. Culture of the excised valve was negative. Following the operation the patient was given a further 10 days' antibiotic therapy with vancomycin and gentamicin.

Chapter 14
Infective Endocarditis

Definition, sites and organisms
Questions

1 Give a definition of 'infective endocarditis'.
2 What is the mortality of infective endocarditis?
3 What is *acute* infective endocarditis? Which organisms are most likely to cause it?
4i What type of person is most likely to develop infective endocarditis? At what sites is it most likely to occur? In what percentage of cases is the disease estimated to occur on a previously normal valve?
  ii Which site within the heart is most likely to be infected in a drug addict?
5i What are the three or four most commonly found infecting organisms in ordinary clinical practice?
  ii With which organism is a drug addict most likely to be infected?
  iii Which organisms are most likely on an artificial valve?
  iv What organisms are most likely to cause culture negative cases?

Answers

1 Definition

Infective endocarditis is defined as a disease caused by dissemination of an infective agent from a focus of infection on a valve or other part of the endocardium of the heart.
Traditionally two forms of infective endocarditis are recognised, acute and subacute. In practice, however, the two forms represent the ends of a continuous spectrum.

2 Mortality

Despite modern antibiotic therapy the mortality of infective endocarditis is 15–30%.

3 Acute infective endocarditis

This is the form of the disease associated with rapid destruction of endocardial tissue as a result of infection with highly virulent organisms such as *Staphylococcus aureus*, *Neisseria gonorrhoeae* or *Streptococcus pneumoniae*.

4 Persons most likely to be infected and the sites of infection

i   Infective endocarditis tends to occur on (a) valves previously damaged by rheumatic fever, (b) bicuspid aortic valves and prolapsing mitral valves, neither of which may have been recognised previously, and (c) at the site of congenital lesions. In about 30% of cases the condition is thought to occur on a previously normal valve. Partly because rheumatic fever is becoming less common, the age of patients with infective endocarditis is increasing.

The commonest site of infection is the aortic valve, then the mitral valve followed by congenital lesions such as ventricular septal defect and unclosed persistent ductus arteriosus. Infection of an atrial septal defect is rare. About 2% of artificial valves become infected.

ii   Because it faces the incoming infected blood and is sited before the lungs, the tricuspid valve is the most likely site of infection in a drug addict.

5 The bacteria causing infective endocarditis

i   *Organisms causing infective endocarditis* tend to be normal commensals from various parts of the body. Infection with *Staphylococcus aureus* may arise from a boil or infected spot on the skin. *Overall 80% of cases are due to infection with streptococci or staphylococci.*
• About 60% of cases are due to *Streptococcus viridans*, a commensal from the mouth.
• The next most common organisms are the group D streptococci, such as *Streptococcus faecalis*, a commensal from the gut or an infecting organism in the urinary tract.

ii   *In drug addicts* 60% of infections are due to *Staphylococcus aureus* the remainder tending to be due to the organisms listed in the next paragraph.

iii   *Artificial valves* are likely to be infected by *Staphylococcus epidermidis*, or Gram negative organisms such as *Bacteroides*, *Escherichia coli* or *Haemophilus influenzae*.

iv   *Most culture negative cases* are due to penicillin sensitive streptococci. Rarely a culture negative case may be due to Q fever caused by *Coxiella burneti*, or a fungus such as *Monilia*.

Symptoms, signs, investigation

Questions

6   List the symptoms and signs of infective endocarditis. What are Osler's nodes and the glomerulonephritis associated with the condition thought to be due to?

7   What investigations would you order in a case of suspected infective endocarditis?

Answers

6   **Symptoms and signs**

The symptoms of the condition were well illustrated by the case of Miss U-R. In almost 100% of cases the patient complains of generalised unwellness, tiredness, and aches and pains. Breathlessness may occur due either to the general unwellness or to cardiac failure.

Signs

● *Fever* occurs at some time in almost all cases, although in about 10% of cases there is no fever at the time of presentation.
● *Cardiac murmurs* occur in over 90% of cases, due either to pre-existing disease or to aortic or mitral regurgitation occurring as a result of destruction of a valve cusp.
● *Clubbing of the finger nails* occurs in 10–50% of cases.
● *Splenomegaly* occurs in about half the cases and is a response to the chronic bacteraemia.
● *Infected arterial emboli* break off from the site of infection in almost a third of cases causing strokes and ischaemia or infarction of gut, kidney, spleen or limb. When infective endocarditis occurs on a congenital lesion with a left to right shunt emboli tend to be swept into the pulmonary circulation causing pleurisy and patchy pneumonia.
● *Osler's nodes* occur in about half the cases and consist of tender red indurated lesions in the pulps of the fingers and toes, lasting a day or so.
● *Splinter haemorrhages* of the finger nails are a non-specific sign that are found frequently in healthy people as a result of trauma, and also in patients with arteritis. Conjunctival splinters are more specific.
● *Petechial haemorrhages* on the neck and chest occur occasionally.
● *Heart failure* occurs in about a third to a half of the cases, and is often in part due to the toxic effects of the infection upon the myocardium as well as to any valvular lesion. Rupture of a valve results in acute heart failure.
● *Other signs* that may occasionally be found include *Janeway lesions*, which are transient non-tender macular patches on the palms and soles, and *Roth spots*, which are haemorrhages with a pale centre in the fundus.
Although they may be due to microemboli, it is possible that Janeway lesions, Roth spots, Osler's nodes and the petechial haemorrhages found in infective endocarditis are due to a form of vasculitis caused by bacterial antigens forming antigen/antibody complexes with the consumption of complement. In support of this it is known that the infective process leads to an intense

immune response with elevated levels of immunoglobulin, and that as well as being affected by septic emboli, the kidney may be affected by immune complexes causing focal and diffuse proliferative glomerulonephritis.

7   Investigation

This was discussed in the answers to Miss U-R's case. In over half the cases the full blood count reveals an anaemia of chronic illness, and the ESR is invariably elevated. The urine contains red blood cells in about 50% of cases. However, as previously stated the two specific investigations are serial blood cultures and echocardiography.

● *Between four and six blood cultures* should be taken over a period of a few hours to a few days, depending upon the urgency with which it is necessary to start treatment. Drug sensitivities and minimum bactericidal concentrations or minimum inhibitory concentrations should be determined. During treatment the bactericidal power of the patient's serum may be measured using the bacteria initially isolated from the patient.

● *Echocardiography* may show thickened valves, sometimes with vegetations.

Treatment
Questions

8   Which drugs are recommended for the treatment of infective endocarditis? What are the dosages and for how long are they given?
9   What are the indications for surgical treatment in infective endocarditis?
10   What antibiotics are used as prophylaxis against infective endocarditis?

Answers

8   The drug treatment of infective endocarditis

This will depend upon the organism that is isolated. The drugs most commonly prescribed are benzylpenicillin, gentamicin and flucloxacillin. In general, the length of the course is determined by the sensitivity of the organism, indicated by the minimum bactericidal or minimum inhibitory concentration of the drug, and the rapidity with which the patient responds.

Drugs are given by intravenous bolus, and not by continuous infusion. The recommended dose of benzylpenicillin is 1.2 g (2 mega units) every 4 hours. The recommended dose of gentamicin is about 1 mg per kilogram body weight every 8 hours, adjusted to give a peak value of 5-10 mg/litre and a trough value < 2 mg/litre. Because of ototoxicity and nephrotoxicity blood levels of gentamicin should be measured twice per week. The recommended dose of flucloxacillin is 2 g every 4 hours.

Patients who are genuinely allergic to penicillin should be given vancomycin 750 mg every 12 hours together with gentamicin, blood levels of both drugs being monitored as the combination is potentially ototoxic.

Specific situations

● *When treatment is necessary whilst isolation is awaited give:* benzylpenicillin and gentamicin.

If the patient is a drug addict or has skin sepsis suggesting infection with *Staphylococcus aureus*, flucloxacillin should be added.

● *Infection due to streptococci:* benzylpenicillin and gentamicin for 2-4 weeks depending upon the minimum bactericidal concentration, followed by oral ampicillin for a further 2-4 weeks.

● *Infection due to Staphylococcus aureus or Staphylococcus epidermidis:* Flucloxacillin 2 g every 4 hours and gentamicin every 8 hours for 2 weeks, followed by flucloxacillin for a further 2-4 weeks.

9   The indications for surgery

Excision of the infected area and its replacement with a prosthesis is recommended for:

● Development or worsening of cardiac failure.
● Resistant organism or failure of the patient to respond to appropriate treatment.
● Increasing aortic or mitral regurgitation.
● Large mobile vegetations on echocardiography.

10   Antibiotic prophylaxis

Although its efficacy is unproven in man, to minimise the risk of bacteraemia following instrumentation, patients known to have rheumatic or congenital heart disease, or an artificial valve should receive:

● Amoxycillin 3 g orally about 1 hour before dentistry.
● Ampicillin 1 g and gentamicin 100 mg, intramuscularly before instrumentation of the gastrointestinal or genitourinary systems.

Those who are genuinely allergic to penicillin may be given erythromycin 500 mg orally before dentistry followed by 500 mg four times a day for 2 days, or a single intravenous dose of vancomycin followed by gentamicin before instrumentation of the gastrointestinal or genitourinary systems.

Further Reading

Braunwald E (ed) (1984). *Heart Disease*, 2nd edition. WB Saunders, Philadelphia. Chapter 32, infective endocarditis.
Weatherall DJ, Ledingham JGG, Warrell DA (eds) (1987). *Oxford Textbook of Medicine*, 2nd edition. Oxford University Press, Oxford. Infective endocarditis, pp 13.314-24.

Case J   More about the Previous Case, the Ill Lady, Miss U-R

On the fifth postoperative day, when she was up and about the ward recovering from the operation at which her infected mitral valve had been replaced by an artificial prosthesis, Miss U-R suddenly developed severe pleuritic pain over the anterior right side of the chest.

Miss U-R's further history

Question

1   What do you think had happened to her?

Answer

1   Pleuritic chest pain after an operation

This suggests a pulmonary embolus, which in Miss U-R's case was confirmed by a spike of temperature, 38°C, and the production of mucoid blood stained sputum. With appropriate treatment she made an uneventful recovery and was discharged home a week later.

Chapter 15
Pulmonary Embolism

Clinical background
Questions

1   Clinically pulmonary embolus is divided into two main syndromes. What are they? What is the important difference between them?

2   From what sites within the body do pulmonary emboli originate? What is the significance of any physical signs in the legs?

3   What was the triad of pathological factors that Virchow recognised as predisposing to the development of venous thrombosis? Bearing these factors in mind, what groups of people are particularly at risk of pulmonary embolism?

4   Which groups of people should be anticoagulated prophylactically to prevent venous thrombosis and pulmonary embolism?

Answers

1   The two main syndromes of pulmonary embolus

● *Acute minor pulmonary embolism* causing pulmonary infarction as a result of an embolus in a peripheral branch of the pulmonary artery.

● *Acute massive pulmonary embolism* due to obstruction of 50% or more of the pulmonary circulation.

The important distinction between the two syndromes is that massive pulmonary embolism is accompanied by profound circulatory effects whereas minor pulmonary embolus has no important effects on the circulation although it may be a harbinger of a subsequent massive pulmonary embolus. Very rarely a syndrome of chronic minor pulmonary embolism may occur, associated with the development of pulmonary hypertension that is unresponsive to treatment.

2   The sites from which pulmonary emboli originate, and the significance of any physical signs in the legs

The great majority of pulmonary emboli arise as a result of dislodgement of thrombus from the deep veins of the legs or pelvis. The factors underlying this are discussed in the answer to the next question. Occasionally pulmonary embolism occurs as a result of dislodgement of a thrombus from the right side of the heart. This may occur with thrombus formation in a fibrillating right atrium or from thrombus that has formed over a myocardial infarct involving the right ventricle. Rarely pulmonary embolism also occurs as a result of a fat or air embolus entering the systemic venous circulation following a fracture, or as the result of amniotic fluid embolus.

It is important to appreciate that in about 50% of cases of deep vein thrombosis of the leg there are no physical signs, and that conversely signs such as tenderness and swelling of the calf and a positive Homans' sign (pain in the calf on flexing the foot) may be present with conditions such as a torn calf muscle as well as venous thrombosis. Such signs are therefore of little diagnostic help.

3 Virchow's triad and the groups of people at particular risk of pulmonary embolism

Virchow's triad of factors predisposing to venous thrombosis are:
- Stasis
- Damage to the vessel wall
- Altered coagulability of the blood

One or more of these factors can usually be identified in the following groups of people at particular risk of venous thrombosis and pulmonary embolism; patients who are ill in bed with medical conditions such as heart failure, myocardial infarction or stroke; those recovering from surgery, particularly the obese and elderly; young women who are pregnant or taking the contraceptive pill; those with varicose veins or a past history of venous thrombosis or pulmonary embolism.

4 Prophylactic anticoagulation

Subcutaneous heparin 5000 units three times per day has been shown to reduce the incidence of venous thrombosis and death from pulmonary embolus when given before, during and after surgery, and is particularly indicated in those aged over 50, those undergoing abdominal or pelvic surgery, those with varicose veins or a past history of venous thrombosis or pulmonary embolism. Many authorities recommend full anticoagulation with warfarin for ill *medical* patients who are confined to bed because of severe myocardial infarction, stroke or the Guillain-Barré syndrome.

Acute minor pulmonary embolism
Questions

5   What are the main clinical features of the condition?
6   How is it investigated? What are the shortcomings of isotope scanning? What is the definitive investigation of this type of pulmonary embolism?
7   How is acute minor pulmonary embolism treated? What does treatment do to the existing infarct?

Answers

5   Clinical features

Small pulmonary emboli may produce no symptoms. Conversely, one or more features of a triad consisting of *breathlessness, haemoptysis and pleuritic chest pain* may occur. The pleuritic chest pain indicates involvement of the pleura. *Wheezing* due to bronchospasm may also occur. Infarction of lung tissue often causes a *spike of pyrexia*, and in an otherwise well patient recovering from an operation an unexplained spike of temperature should arouse suspicion of pulmonary emboli.

On examination there may be a pleural rub or crackles at the site of infarction or signs of pleural effusion.

6   Investigation

● Although plain chest x-ray is normal in about half the cases, in the remainder pulmonary emboli produce small shadows that are typically at the base of the lung, and often linear. In addition a pleural effusion may be seen as a result of the pleural reaction caused by the embolus.

● *Ventilation/perfusion scanning* may be performed using two isotopes, one inhaled, the other injected intravenously to look for differences in the ventilation and perfusion of the lung. A normal perfusion scan excludes a pulmonary embolus. An abnormality on the perfusion scan may be due either to a pulmonary embolus or to a lung condition that affects the pulmonary circulation, such as emphysema. The ventilation scan helps to elucidate this. When a *large* lesion is seen on the perfusion scan and the ventilation scan is normal a pulmonary embolus is highly likely; when both are abnormal a disorder of the lung such as emphysema is likely. However, it is important to appreciate the limitations of ventilation/perfusion scanning. A *small* perfusion defect in the presence of a normal ventilation scan may in fact be due to a lesion other than a pulmonary embolus, whilst a defect on both the perfusion and the ventilation scans may occasionally be due to a pulmonary embolus that has affected ventilation as well as perfusion.

● *Pulmonary angiography.* Because of the difficulties in interpreting isotope scans the definitive test for the diagnosis of pulmonary embolus is finding a filling defect when contrast medium is injected into the pulmonary circulation. However, the test is invasive, but should be available in most large hospitals.

7   Treatment

Anticoagulation reduces the mortality of untreated pulmonary embolus from about a third to about 5%. An intravenous infusion of heparin, usually about 30000 units per day adjusted according to the partial thromboplastin time, should be given for 2 or 3 days until warfarin administered orally at the same time has an effect.

However, it is important to appreciate that heparin and warfarin are given as prophylaxis against extension of the venous thrombosis and further emboli, and do not lyse established emboli, recovery from which depends upon naturally occurring thrombolysis.

Warfarin, monitored regularly to keep the prothrombin ratio between 2½ and 3½, is continued for 3-6 months.

Acute massive pulmonary embolism

Questions

8   What are the main clinical features of the condition?
9   What is the main differential diagnosis of acute massive pulmonary embolus?
10   How is it investigated?
11   How is it treated?

Answers

8   Clinical features

• Acute massive pulmonary embolism obstructs the outflow tract from the right ventricle causing reduction of cardiac output and circulatory collapse. The main clinical features are therefore a triad consisting of *collapse with acute right heart failure, shock and breathlessness*.

• As a consequence of the right heart failure, the central venous pressure rises causing elevation of the jugular venous pulse and dilatation of the thin walled right ventricle, and usually an associated third and possibly a fourth heart sound. Because the dilated right ventricle requires more time to empty than the left ventricle, closure of the pulmonary valve is delayed causing wide splitting of the second heart sound.

• In addition, in about a third of patients dissemination of the embolus to the periphery results in haemoptysis and pleuritic chest pain. A third of patients also complain of angina-like pain that may be mistaken for the pain of myocardial infarction.

9   Differential diagnosis

This is from other causes of acute collapse such as septicaemic shock, myocardial infarction and rupture of the aorta, oesophagus or an abdominal organ. The most useful differentiating signs are the elevated central venous pressure, and the changes in the heart sounds.

10   Investigation

• The definitive tests are isotope scanning and pulmonary angiography, both of which have ben described.
• *Blood gases*. Typically the PaO_2 is low due to failure of oxygenation of the blood and the $PaCO_2$ is low due to the air hunger and hyperventilation that accompanies the condition.

- *Chest x-ray* may show reduced pulmonary markings in affected areas due to reduced blood flow. In addition the right or left pulmonary arteries may appear abruptly cut off at the site of occlusion.
- *Electrocardiograph* may be normal or show changes of right ventricular strain, most commonly a deep S wave in lead I due to the abnormally large electrical impulse produced by the right ventricle travelling away from that lead. A Q wave and T wave inversion also occur in lead III giving rise to the so-called S_1, Q_3, T_3 pattern. In addition the T wave may be inverted in the chest leads over the right ventricle, namely leads V_1-V_3. Right bundle branch block may also occur.

11   Treatment

This is with oxygen and either intravenous heparin, intravenous streptokinase or tissue plasminogen activator or urokinase, or by surgical pulmonary embolectomy. Unlike heparin, streptokinase, tissue plasminogen activator and urokinase cause lysis of the embolus and are probably as effective as embolectomy. A reasonable strategem is therefore to prescribe streptokinase or tissue plasminogen activator, unless contraindicated by a tendency to bleed, reserving embolectomy for patients in whom the drugs are contraindicated or those whose condition deteriorates despite an hour or so of the drugs.

Once the acute phase has passed, conventional anticoagulant treatment with warfarin should be instigated and continued for 3-6 months.

Further Reading

Weatherall DJ, Ledingham JGG, Warrell DA (eds) (1987). *Oxford Textbook of Medicine*, 2nd edition. Oxford University Press, Oxford. Pulmonary embolism, pp 13.355-60.

Cases K-N Four Cases of Breathlessness due to Respiratory Disease

Breathlessness: classification of causes
Question

1   Before proceeding to the first case, list the commoner causes of breathlessness due to both respiratory disease and other causes, classifying them according to underlying mechanism.

Answer

1   Causes of breathlessness

Our lack of knowledge about the way the sensation of breathlessness is produced is discussed on page 7. As suggested there, at the present time the most attractive hypothesis is that breathlessness occurs when the tension developed by the respiratory muscles is excessive in relation to their movement. With this in mind the causes of breathlessness may be classified by underlying mechanism as follows:

Physiological

●   Exertion—causing increased work by the respiratory muscles.

Psychological

●   Fear or fright—causing increased cortical drive.
●   Hyperventilation—either due to increased conscious or unconscious cortical drive.

Obstructive airways disease

●   Asthma, chronic bronchitis and emphysema causing:
a   increased work by the respiratory muscles,
b   in severe cases, anoxia resulting from mismatching of ventilation and perfusion.

Anoxia stimulating the carotid and aortic body chemoreceptors:

●   High altitude
●   *Mismatching of ventilation and perfusion of the lung.*
Normally ventilation and perfusion of the lungs match one another in such a way as to ensure optimum exchange of oxygen and carbon dioxide between alveoli and pulmonary capillaries. However, in many diseases there is an important element of

mismatching of these parameters which if severe enough may result in anoxia that may contribute to the breathlessness of the condition. Examples are:

a   Pneumonia
b   Pulmonary embolus
c   Carcinoma of the bronchus
d   Asthma, emphysema, chronic bronchitis
e   Pulmonary fibrosis
f   Pulmonary congestion

Restrictive disease

● *Restrictive lung disease* such as pulmonary fibrosis of any cause, pulmonary oedema, or pneumonia:
a   rendering the lung stiff and increasing the work of the respiratory muscles,
b   causing mismatching of ventilation and perfusion,
c   interfering with diffusion of gases across the alveolar-capillary membrane.
● *Restricted movement of the chest wall* due to conditions such as:
a   pain from a fractured rib or pleurisy,
b   conditions of the thoracic skeleton such as ankylosing spondylitis,
c   neuropathy affecting the respiratory muscles, for example polio or the Guillain-Barré syndrome.
● *Pleural effusion of any cause* resulting in:
a   increased work by the respiratory muscles,
b   increased stimulation of the respiratory centre by vagal afferents from the lung collapsed by the effusion.

Pulmonary congestion

This causes stiffness of the lung and an increase in the work of the respiratory muscles, and in severe cases, mismatching of ventilation and perfusion, and impaired diffusion of gases across the alveolar-capillary membrane. Examples are:
● Left ventricular failure
● Pulmonary oedema due to other causes such as mitral stenosis

Metabolic

● *Acidosis*, due for example to renal failure or diabetic ketoacidosis, resulting in H^+ ions stimulating the respiratory centre, although in practice only occasional patients with Kussmaul's deep sighing acidotic breathing complain of breathlessness.
● *Severe anaemia*. The degree of anaemia causing breathlessness varies but is often about Hb 6–8 g%.

NOTE: As implied in some of the preceding examples, many conditions cause breathlessness as a result of a combination of several of the above mechanisms. Thus carcinoma of the lung may affect ventilation/perfusion, cause a pleural effusion or limit movement of the chest wall because of pain. Left ventricular failure may cause congestion of the lungs rendering them stiff and non-compliant thus increasing the work of ventilation, and in severe cases may also cause abnormal ventilation/perfusion, impaired diffusion of gases through frank pulmonary oedema, or restriction due to pleural effusion.

Case K

Case No. 1: Miss L-A, aged 20 years

A shorthand typist living at home with her parents.

History of present condition

Referred by her family doctor with a history of having been intermittently chesty and breathless since infancy, and wheezing after running about 100 yards. The specific reason for her referral was that during the previous week she had suddenly come over very breathless and blue and had lost consciousness when cleaning up after an evening dog training class. She had never smoked and did not cough any sputum.

Examination

A well looking young woman in whom clinical examination was normal. BP 120/70 lying and standing. Spirometry, FEV$_1$/VC = 3.2/3.8 (84%).

Miss L-A

Questions

1   What diagnosis is suggested by the history?
2   Miss L-A's spirometry was FEV$_1$/VC = 3.2/3.8 (84%).
i   Define the terms FEV$_1$ and VC.
ii   What are the three patterns of results spirometry may yield and in which disease processes is each abnormal pattern seen?
iii   Interpret the following results:

	FEV$_1$	VC	%	Predicted FEV$_1$/VC
(a) Middle-aged man	0.6	1.8	33	4.0/5.0
(b) Middle-aged man	1.8	4.0	45	4.0/5.0
(c) Middle-aged man	1.3	1.6	81	4.0/5.0
(d) Miss L-A	3.2	3.8	84	3.5/4.0

3i   What is peak expiratory flow rate (PEFR)? How is it measured? Upon what factors does it depend?
ii   What are the advantages and disadvantages of peak flow measurements compared with measurements made by spirometer?

Answers

1   The diagnosis in Miss L-A's case

With the exception of rare disorders like cystic fibrosis, most chesty children are suffering from asthma (discussed on page 229). In Miss L-A's case this suggestion is supported by the history of wheezing with exercise and breathlessness leading to unconsciousness on exposure to dogs.

2   Spirometry

i   Spirometry involves timing and measuring the volume of a fast forced expiration from the top of inspiration when the lungs are at total lung capacity (TLC) to the bottom of expiration. The amount of air expired in the first second is known as the forced expiratory volume in one second or FEV_1, and is related to the force generated by the expiratory muscles and the width of the airways. The total volume of air blown out from the top of inspiration to the bottom of expiration is known as the vital capacity, VC. The volume of air remaining in the lungs at the bottom of expiration is known as the residual volume, RV.

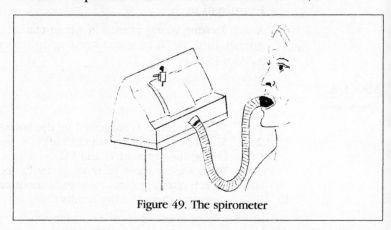

Figure 49. The spirometer

ii   The three patterns of results of spirometry, and the disease processes associated with the abnormal patterns are:
●   *Normal*. In this situation the vital capacity is normal for the height and age of the subject who is able to blow out 70% or more of their vital capacity in one second, i.e. $FEV_1/VC > 70\%$.
●   *Obstructive*. In this situation, because the airways are narrow, expiration takes longer than normal. The volume of air exhaled in the first second is therefore small, resulting in FEV_1/VC less than 70%. Obstructive results are obtained in chronic obstructive airways disease due either to chronic bronchitis or emphysema, during an attack of asthma, and occasionally with pulmonary oedema, presumably because of spasm and oedema of the airways.
●   *Restrictive*. In this situation movement of the thorax is limited by either stiffness of the lungs or skeletal problems that

prevent full inspiration and expiration, although there is no obstruction of the airways. As a result of limited movement of the thorax, the vital capacity is small although because there is no obstruction the patient easily expires what vital capacity there is. Thus despite a small vital capacity, $FEV_1/VC > 70\%$.

The main causes of restrictive results are:

a   *Skeletal conditions* such as ankylosing spondylitis, fractured rib, pleurisy and kyphosis.

b   *Neurological conditions* that result in impaired movement of the thorax, such as the Guillain–Barré syndrome.

c   *Stiff lungs* due to conditions such as pulmonary fibrosis or pulmonary oedema, due for instance, to left ventricular failure.

d   *Pleural effusion.*

iii   Interpretation of results:

	FEV_1	VC	%	Interpretation
(a) Middle-aged man	0.6	1.8	33	Severe obstruction
(b) Middle-aged man	1.8	4.0	45	Moderate obstruction
(c) Middle-aged man	1.3	1.6	81	Severe restriction*
(d) Miss L-A	3.2	3.8	84	Normal

* This pattern may also occur with severe obstruction as a result of the airways closing as expiration proceeds.

●   Because it gives so much information about the diagnosis and severity of a disease, spirometry should be performed in all breathless patients with the possible exception of those whose dyspnoea is clearly due to non-respiratory causes such as cardiac failure or anaemia.

3   Peak expiratory flow rate (PEFR)

i   PEFR is the highest flow rate that is achieved when forced expiration is begun with the lungs full at total lung capacity. It is

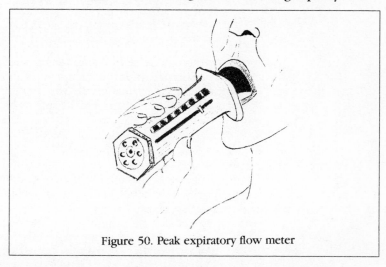

Figure 50. Peak expiratory flow meter

measured by getting the patient to inhale fully and blow out as hard and fast as possible through a small handheld meter. Again the result depends upon the force generated by the expiratory muscles and the width of the airways. Peak flow occurs about 10 milliseconds after the beginning of expiration.

ii

● *The advantage* of the peak flow meter is that it is small and mobile, making it easy to obtain repeated measurements.
● *The disadvantage* is that it gives only a crude overall measure of ventilatory capacity without the facility provided by the spirometer for discriminating between the various pathological patterns.

Cases K-N Cases Nos. 2-4

Question

1   Read the following three cases histories and make a diagnosis of the cause of the breathlessness in each case. In each instance, comment on the results of the spirometry.

Case No. 2: Mr L-C, aged 65 years

An unmarried retail pharmacist known to suffer from coeliac disease (gluten enteropathy).

History of present condition

About 6 months prior to attending the clinic, this man developed a summer cold followed by daily attacks of wheezing, growling chest and breathlessness. His condition was almost completely relieved for a few hours by inhalation of salbutamol he had obtained for himself from his shop. He had never smoked, did not cough any sputum and denied any past or family history of allergy, asthma, eczema or hay fever.

Past medical history

Apart from coeliac disease, for about 5 years he had been taking atenolol for hypertension.

Examination

A well looking late middle-aged man in whom clinical examination was normal except for reduced breath sounds and slightly prolonged expiration. BP 190/100 lying and standing. Spirometry, $FEV_1/VC = 1.4/2.5$ (56%).

Case No. 3:
Mrs J-L, aged 66 years

A widowed retired shorthand typist living alone in her own bungalow.

History of present condition

For 14 years this lady had experienced increasing shortness of breath, mainly on exertion, but also for the first 2 hours after waking in the morning, and at times in the winter. Her exercise tolerance was limited to 200 yards on the flat. Because of breathlessness she was obliged to sleep supported by three pillows. She had smoked 15 cigarettes per day until 10 years previously. She coughed white or occasionally green sputum throughout the year.

Past medical history

Left nephrectomy for hydronephrosis 10 years previously. Hypertension suspected 14 years previously, but not treated.

Examination

A thin middle-aged lady in whom clinical examination was normal except for slight central cyanosis, bilaterally reduced breath sounds and a few early crackles at the base of the left lung. BP 160/90 lying and standing. Spirometry, $FEV_1/VC = 0.4/1.0$ (40%).

Case No. 4:
Mrs I-A, aged 65 years

A widowed lady living alone in her own second floor flat to which she could gain access only by struggling up 28 stairs.

History of present condition

The first time this lady had been seen was 2 years previously when she had presented with chest pain that was worse with coughing, stretching and opposing the muscles of the arms, and was clearly of musculoskeletal origin. The nature of this had been explained to her and she had been reassured and discharged. However, at that time she had also complained of breathlessness on exertion. Because no cause for this, such as heart failure or airways obstruction, was immediately obvious, it had been ascribed to anxiety.

On this occasion she had been referred back to the clinic because of a dry cough and breathlessness that had increased to a point where she was short of breath walking about her flat.

Specific direct questions

The answers to these were all negative. She had never smoked and denied any past personal or family history of allergy, asthma, eczema, hayfever or particular time of the day or year when her breathlessness was worse. She had not been exposed to any dusts and did not keep birds.

Examination

A small middle-aged lady with marked cyanosis of the lips, tongue and periphery, and a tendency to pant on minimal exertion. The fingers were grossly clubbed and there were 'showers' of coarse late inspiratory crackles at the lung bases. Otherwise clinical examination was normal. BP 140/80 lying and standing. Spirometry, $FEV_1/VC = 1.4/1.6$ (87%).

Answers

1   Diagnosis of Cases Nos. 2–4

Case No. 2: Mr L-C

The history of wheeze and breathlessness starting with a chest infection in an adult is suggestive of intrinsic or non-allergic asthma. This is fully discussed on page 238. About half of the people suffering with this type of asthma give a history of the condition starting at the time of a respiratory tract infection. The diagnosis is supported by the response to salbutamol, the obstructive results of spirometry and the lack of evidence of other conditions such as heart failure.

Case No. 3: Mrs J-L

The history of breathlessness on exertion for 14 years, particularly on rising in the morning and in the winter, together with heavy smoking, a chronic cough productive of sputum, reduced breath sounds, and very obstructive spirometry all suggest that Mrs J-L was suffering from chronic obstructive lung disease. This is discussed on page 248.

Case No. 4: Mrs L-A

The occurrence of (a) breathlessness with a dry non-productive cough, (b) clubbing of the fingers and (c) late bilateral inspiratory crackles in a patient who denies exposure to dusts constitutes a triad that should always suggest the likelihood of cryptogenic fibrosing alveolitis. This suggestion is supported by the restrictive results of spirometry and is discussed on page 269.

Comments about Cases Nos. 2–4
Questions

2   Comment on the appropriateness or otherwise of the atenolol Mr L-C, Case No. 2, was taking.
3   What type of drug is salbutamol? What is its mode of action? What diseases it is used to treat?

Answers

2   **The significance of the atenolol Mr L-C was taking**

Atenolol is a beta blocking drug. Although it is said to be cardioselective, blocking mainly ß1 adrenoreceptors, to a lesser extent it may also block the bronchodilator ß2 adrenoreceptors to bronchial smooth muscle, and as discussed on page 100, may precipitate severe or even fatal asthma.

Changing Mr L-C's hypotensive treatment from atenolol to the calcium channel blocking drug, nifedipine, led to a slight improvement in his condition, although eventually a short course of oral steroids was needed to restore his breathing to normal.

3   **Salbutamol**

Salbutamol is a ß2 and to a slight extent a ß1 adrenergic agonist that mimics the beta actions of adrenaline. Therapeutically its main actions are to cause relaxation of bronchial smooth muscle and stabilisation of mast cells. Within the cell it is thought to activate the enzyme adenyl cyclase leading to an increase of cAMP.

Salbutamol is used in the treatment of asthma and those cases of chronic obstructive airways disease in which there is a reversible component.

Chapter 16
Asthma

Definition and incidence

Questions

1   Define the term 'bronchial asthma'.
2   Define the terms 'incidence' and 'prelavence'. What is the prevalence of asthma in the population? What is its sex distribution? What is the natural history of most cases of childhood asthma?

Answers

1   Definition of bronchial asthma

● *Introduction*. For the convenience of study and thinking, three patterns of airways obstruction or airways limitation are traditionally recognised, namely asthma, chronic bronchitis and emphysema. Often these are easily recognisable clinical entities. However, it is important to appreciate that in many instances they tend to overlap and are difficult to separate. For instance, most patients with chronic airways obstruction have *both* emphysema and chronic bronchitis. Some have a reversible or 'asthmatic' component, whilst at the other end of the spectrum, particularly if they smoke, some true asthmatics go on to develop irreversible disease similar to chronic obstructive airways disease. For these reasons, to minimise arguments about definitions and characterisation it is probably best to think of the three conditions as a continuum from variable airways obstruction due to allergy at one end of the spectrum, to smoking related irreversible chronic obstructive airways disease at the other.
● *Definition of bronchial asthma*. With the above limitations in mind, bronchial asthma may be defined as *episodic* breathlessness, wheeze or tightness of the chest due to hyperactivity of the bronchial tree causing reversible airways obstruction. Asthma may be caused by a wide variety of stimuli.

NOTE: Bronchial asthma must not be confused with cardiac asthma, a term used to describe breathlessness due to pulmonary oedema resulting from left ventricular failure.

2   Definition of the terms incidence and prevalence. The prevalence of asthma, its sex distribution, and the natural history of most cases of childhood asthma

● *Incidence* is the *annual rate* of occurrence within a population of a condition or phenomenon. *Prevalence* is the *total amount* of a condition or phenomenon within a population, that is the summation of annual incidences less those in whom the condition has resolved.

● The prevalence of asthma varies according to the criteria used to define it. Using wheeze as the defining term, about 10% of children and about 5% of adults may be classified as asthmatic. On the other hand, using episodic breathlessness as the defining term, the usually quoted figures for asthma are about 2% of the population in the United Kingdom and about 3% of the population in the United States.

● During childhood twice as many boys as girls are affected by asthma. However, this gradually changes so that for adults the prevalence is about the same in both sexes.

● Remission occurs in about 75% of cases of childhood asthma. However, there is a high probability of relapse in middle age, particularly among those who wheeze occasionally during adult life.

Airways obstruction in asthma
Question

3   Obstruction of the airways in asthma is caused by three main factors.
i   Contraction of bronchial smooth muscle is one of them. What are the other two?
ii   What effects do the three combined have on the mechanics of the lung?

Answer

3   Causes and effects of airways obstruction

i   The three main factors causing airways obstruction in asthma are:
● Contraction of bronchial smooth muscle.
● Oedema and inflammation of the bronchial mucosa.
● Mucus plugs obstructing the airways.

ii   Their combined effect upon the mechanics of the lung may be summarised as:
● *Increased work of breathing.* Because of the increased resistance to flow of air along the narrowed airways the patient has to breathe harder resulting in the respiratory muscles using more oxygen and energy than normal.
● *Mismatching of ventilation and perfusion.* Normally ventilation and perfusion of the lungs match each other in such a way as to ensure optimum exchange of oxygen and carbon dioxide

between the alveoli and caapillaries. However, in asthma both ventilation and perfusion may be adversely affected, obstruction of airways, for instance, resulting in failure of ventilation of some alveoli and perfusion without ventilation.

● *Reduction of the lung's elastic recoil.* Asthma is associated with trapping of air in the periphery of the lung causing it to become hyper-inflated and stretched. Stretching of the lung's elastin fibres impairs its elastic recoil and contributes to the increased work of breathing. This is more fully explained on page 251.

Humoral and neurological mechanisms (i)
Question

4i   Which cells are classically described as being involved in the release of humoral meditators during an attack of allergic asthma?

ii   List the substances released via or by these cells during an attack of allergic asthma. Write notes about the substances thought to be involved in the asthmatic process.

iii   What is thought to be the role of eosinophils in the allergic reaction?

Answer

4   The cells and humoral mediators involved in allergic asthma. The role of the eosinophil

i   *Mast cells* are the cells that are thought to be activated to release humoral mediators during an attack of allergic asthma.

ii   *The substances released* may be divided into those that are preformed and stored in granules within the cell, and those that are not stored, but are manufactured at the time of release. The two groups may be summarised as follows:

Preformed stored mediators

Mediators not stored. Manufactured at the time of release

Involved in the asthmatic process:

● Histamine
● Platelet activating factor (PAF)
● Neutrophil chemotactic factor (NCF)   ● Leukotrienes
● Eosinophil chemotactic factor (ECF)   ● Prostaglandin D_2 (PGD_2)
● Proteases

Not involved in the asthmatic process:

● Heparin

● *Histamine.* The physiological role of histamine is uncertain although it is thought to be a neurotransmitter and is known to stimulate gastric acid secretion. Pathologically, it is involved in the inflammatory process, anaphylaxis, and allergic reactions. In asthma it is thought to cause oedema of the bronchial wall and contraction of bronchial smooth muscle.

● *Platelet activating factor (PAF)*. This is a phospholipid released from inflammatory cells, and may have an important role in the asthmatic process. Although its precise mode of action is not clear, it is thought to act indirectly by releasing an as yet unidentified mediator from activated platelets causing:

a   Immediate constriction of bronchial smooth muscle and an increase in the permeability of the bronchial vasculature that results in bronchial oedema.

b   An increase in background hyperactivity of the bronchial tree to other stimuli for up to 4 weeks.

● *The leukotrienes and prostaglandins*. These are substances derived from arachidonic acid, and act as local biological modulators in the tissues in which they are formed. Arachidonic acid is a 20-carbon unsaturated fatty acid derived from a phospholipid in the cell membrane by the action of the enzyme phospholipase.

As shown diagrammatically in the answer to question 5, the leukotrienes are derived from arachidonic acid by the action of the enzyme, *lipoxygenase*, and the prostaglandins by the action of the enzyme, *cycloxygenase*.

a   *The leukotrienes*. The suffix 4 refers to the number of double bonds in the leukotriene molecule. Leukotriene A$_4$ is an unstable intermediate product. Leukotrienes C$_4$, D$_4$ and E$_4$ constitute what was previously known as slow reacting substance of anaphylaxis (SRS-A), and molecule for molecule as bronchoconstrictors are 1000 times as powerful as histamine or the prostaglandins.

Leukotriene B$_4$ is strongly chemotactic for eosinophils and neutrophils and thus contributes to the inflammatory process.

b   *The prostaglandins*. The suffix 2 refers to the number of double bonds in the prostaglandin molecule. The main prostaglandin of the mast cell is PGD$_2$, the function of which is unclear at the present time. Other prostaglandins produced by non-mast cells have better identified actions. These may be summarised as:

PGE$_2$: bronchodilator/vasodilator.

PGF$_2$: bronchoconstrictor/vasoconstrictor.

PG1$_2$ (prostacyclin) formed by vascular endothelium: vasodilator/ inhibitor of platelet aggregation.

TXA$_2$ (thromboxane A$_2$) formed by platelets: platelet aggregator.

● *Neutrophil and eosinophil chemotactic factors*. These are thought to cause an influx of leucocytes into the bronchial wall to participate in the inflammatory reaction.

● *Proteases*. One of the actions of these enzymes is to cause bradykinin, a peptide with bronchoconstrictor effects, to be broken off the plasma protein, kininogen.

iii   *The role of the eosinophil in allergic reactions:* the eosinophil produces tissue damaging substances such as major basic protein (MBP) which probably acts by ionically disrupting cell membranes, eosinophil cationic protein (ECP) and oxygen radicals. In asthma these substances contribute to the inflammatory process and probably increase the permeability of the bronchial mucosa to allergens. In parasitic infections, eosinophils gather round the parasite and attack it with these substances.

Humoral and neurological mechanisms (ii)
Questions

5   Draw a simple diagram using names, not chemical formulae, to show the derivation and relationship of the prostaglandins and leukotrienes to arachidonic acid.

6   Describe the immune process by which the cells that contain the humoral mediators are thought to be activated to release their contents during an attack of allergic asthma.

7   The mechanism by which intrinsic or non-allergic asthma is caused is unknown. What are the main theories that have been advanced to explain it?

Answers

5   Diagram showing the relationship of the prostaglandins and leukotrienes to arachidonic acid

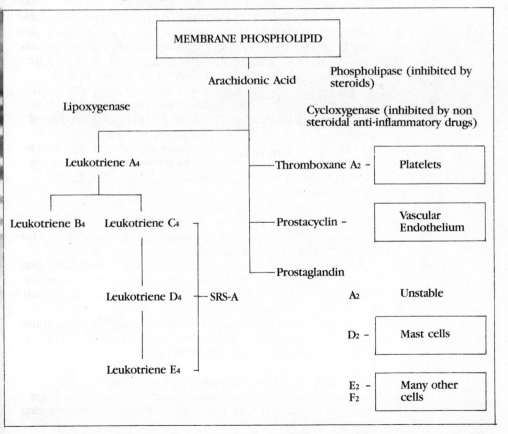

6   The mechanism by which mast cells are thought to release their contents during an attack of asthma

The mechanism by which mast cells are activated to release their contents in allergic asthma occurs in two phases.

●   In the first phase exposure to antigen, or allergen as it is often known in this situation, results in a hypersensitive state in which specific B lymphocytes are activated to mature into plasma cells that produce abnormal amounts of IgE specific to the allergen. Much of this IgE combines with the patient's mast cells rendering them abnormally sensitive to further exposure to the allergen.

●   In the second phase further exposure to the allergen results in activation of the mast cells to release their contents. As shown in Figure 51 this happens in response to bridging of two molecules of IgE attached to the cell by one molecule of allergen.

Hypersensitivity reactions involving IgE and the activation of mast cells occur rapidly within a period of seconds or up to 10-15 minutes of exposure to the antigen, and are therefore known as

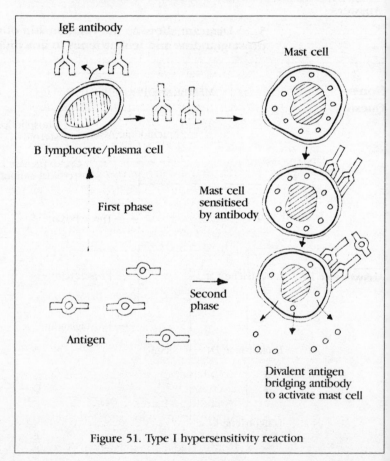

Figure 51. Type I hypersensitivity reaction

immediate or type I hypersensitivity reactions. Typical examples of type I hypersensitivity reactions are allergic asthma, hay fever, atopic dermatitis (eczema), urticaria and anaphylaxis.

7   Theories about the mechanism causing intrinsic asthma

Although a great deal is known about the mechanisms by which extrinsic asthma is caused, very little is known at the present time about the mechanism underlying intrinsic asthma. At least three theories have been advanced to explain it. These involve:

● *The vagus nerve.* The vagus nerve to the lung contains a reflex arc of sensory fibres that are stimulated by irritant stimuli and run centrally to the brain, and motor fibres that affect constriction of bronchial smooth muscle. According to this hypothesis intrinsic asthma is due to activation of this reflex arc.

● *Non-allergic activation of mast cells.* This theory suggests that mast cells are activated by as yet unidentified stimuli.

● *Non-mast cell prostaglandins.* Prostaglandin D_2 is the main prostaglandin of the mast cell. However, other cells within the lungs also manufacture considerable amounts of the bronchodilator prostaglandin, PGE_2, and the bronchoconstrictor prostaglandin, PGF_2. Imbalance of these prostaglandins could be important in the mechanism of intrinsic asthma.

Non-specific triggers; occupational asthma
Questions

8   Apart from specific allergens, attacks of asthma may be precipitated in many asthmatics by several so-called non-specific triggers.

i   List the more common non-specific triggers of asthma.

ii   How are firstly exercise, secondly non-steroidal anti-inflammatory drugs, and thirdly beta blocking drugs thought to precipitate attacks?

9i   List the commoner causes of industrial/occupational asthma.

ii   By what mechanisms is this type of asthma thought to occur?

Answers

8   Non-specific triggers of asthma

i   Whereas allergens provoke asthma only in persons who are allergic to them, several stimuli non-specifically provoke narrowing of the airways in many patients with either allergic or non-allergic asthma. These stimuli are:

● Respiratory tract infection (usually viral)
● Exercise
● Psychological stress
● Atmospheric pollutants such as cigarette smoke and sulphur dioxide
● Non-steroidal anti-inflammatory drugs
● Beta blocking drugs

The mechanisms by which most of these triggers provoke bronchial constriction are unclear although various hypotheses have been advanced to explain them including release of humoral mediators and stimulation of the vagal reflex arc.

ii

● *Exercise*. This is particularly likely to provoke asthma in cold dry air and is due to loss of heat from the bronchial tree, although as implied above, precisely how this causes bronchial constriction is not clear. Exercise per se is not responsible, as asthma does not occur when exercise is performed in warm moist conditions.

● *Analgesics such as aspirin and the other non-steroidal anti-inflammatory drugs*. These provoke attacks of asthma in about 5–10% of asthmatic patients. Reactions are particularly likely in patients with nasal polyps, and occasionally may be so severe as to be fatal. In susceptible individuals the mechanism causing the reaction is probably blocking of the enzyme, cycloxygenase. Two results might follow:

a   The metabolism of arachidonic acid might be diverted towards the powerful bronchoconstrictor leukotriene pathway, and/or

b   The formation of bronchodilator prostaglandin E_2 might be inhibited.

● *Beta blocking drugs*. These may precipitate asthma by competing for and blocking $ß_2$ bronchodilator adrenoreceptors in the lung. This is more fully discussed on page 100.

9   The commoner causes of occupational asthma, and the mechanisms by which they are thought to be caused

i   *The main agents causing occupational asthma* may be summarised as:

● Platinum used for platinum refining.
● Resins used in solders and glues.
● Isocyanates used in paints and plastics.
● Flour and grains used in baking.
● Proteolytic enzymes in detergents.
● Wood dusts created during carpentry.

ii   *At least three mechanisms* are known to be involved in the causation of occupational asthma.

● *Type I hypersensitivity* involving specific IgE antibodies directed against the agent. This is more common in atopic individuals, but also occurs in non-atopic individuals.

● *Type III hypersensitivity* involving the activation of specific IgG antibodies directed against the agent. Reactions of this type involve activation of complement which in turn stimulates a number of reactions that include contraction of smooth muscle by a direct effect, release of kinins from plasma kininogen, and activation of mast cells.

Whereas type I reactions occur within 10–15 minutes of exposure to the agent, type III reactions are delayed by some 3–5

hours and may occur after the individual has left work.
● *Irritation and stimulation of the vagal reflex arc.* An
explanation of this is given in the answer to question 7 on
page 235.

In all cases of occupational asthma the clue to the cause is
provided by the absence of attacks when the individual is away
from work at weekends or on vacation.

The two main clinical types of asthma and the main symptoms of the disease
Questions

10i Traditionally asthma is divided into two clinical types. What
are they? List the factors such as the presence or absence of family
history and allergy that characterise each.
   ii Define the term 'atopy'.
11 List the four main symptoms of asthma.
12 Making a correct diagnosis is often facilitated by knowing
what direct questions to ask. A simple way of thinking about this is
to pretend to 'put on a hat' about the disease or system suspected
of being involved and to ask a list of prepared questions about it.
In the present instance:
   i Using the information contained in the answers to 10 and
11 put on your 'asthma hat' and list the *specific* direct questions
that should be asked in a case of suspected asthma.
   ii Whilst answering this question, put on your 'bronchitis hat'
and list the *specific* direct questions that should be asked in a case
of suspected chronic obstructive airways disease (the term used to
embrace both chronic bronchitis and emphysema).

Answers

10 The clinical types of asthma and the definition of 'atopy'

i Subject to an appreciation that the division of asthma or any
disease into different categories is an artificially created aid to
thinking into which some patients do not fit, the condition is
traditionally divided into two types, namely *extrinsic asthma*, in
which attacks can be precipitated by an external allergen such as
pollen, dust of the house mite or animal dander, and *intrinsic
asthma*, in which no obvious external allergic trigger is
demonstrable. The characteristics of each type are as follows:

Extrinsic asthma

● Usually this type of asthma begins in infancy or childhood,
attacks often being precipitated by a cold. At this stage twice as
many boys as girls are affected.
● In about 50% of cases it is associated with hay fever and/or
eczema (but in about 50% of cases it is not).
● In about 50% of cases there is a *family history* of asthma,
eczema or hay fever (but in 50% of cases there is not).

● *Frequently it is seasonal*. However, it may be non-seasonal in those who are continuously exposed to ubiquitous allergens such as house dust mite.

● Although as discussed in the answer to question 13, they are not usually indicated these days, if done a multiplicity of skin prick tests and bronchial provocation tests are usually positive.

● In keeping with the allergic state of the individual, serum levels of IgE antibody are raised, attacks of asthma being precipitated by the mechanisms described in the answers to questions 4–6.

● There is a 75% chance of the condition remitting during the patient's late teens, although there is a high probability of relapse in middle age, particularly among those who wheeze occasionally during adult life.

Intrinsic asthma

● In this type of asthma no external allergic triggers are demonstrable. Possible mechanisms causing the condition are discussed in the answer to question 7.

● Usually the condition starts after age 30, and affects men and women equally.

● In about 50% of cases the first attack is associated with a respiratory tract infection or flu-like illness.

● Typically there is no personal or family history of other allergic conditions such as asthma, eczema or hay fever, although as previously described, some patients grow out of childhood asthma only to develop asthma again later in life.

● Serum IgE antibody levels are normal, and if done, prick skin tests and bronchial provocation tests are negative.

● Unlike extrinsic asthma, remission is rare, the course usually being chronic and recurrent, not infrequently merging into irreversible disabling chronic obstructive airways disease.

ii   *Atopy* is defined as a familial tendency to asthma, hay fever, eczema or urticaria, or a combination of these conditions. However, as these conditions also occur in persons without a family history, the term tends to be used for the conditions whether or not there is a family history.

11   The four main symptoms of asthma

These tend to be intermittent and are:

● *Cough*. Often productive of tenacious mucus. On the other hand a persistent dry cough may be the only symptom of early asthma.

● *Wheeze*. A description of this sign and the mechanism underlying it is given on page 25.

● *Breathlessness*. Often this wakes the patient in the night, and is particularly noticeable on rising in the morning, as well of course, as during the day.

● *Tightness in the chest*.

12   'Asthma hat' and 'bronchitis hat' questions

i   *Asthma*. These relate to (a) the airways lability that is the hallmark of asthma, and (b) history of allergy. In any patient suspected of suffering from asthma always ask specifically about:

● *Reversibility?* Are there times when the breathing is normal and other times when it is not?

● *Wheeze?* One of the four main symptoms of asthma.

● *Time of day* when the breathing is worse? Discussed below.

● *Time of year* when the breathing is worse? In general, a pattern of breathlessness in the spring and summer is suggestive of asthma, whilst a pattern of breathlessness in the winter is suggestive of chronic obstructive airways disease.

● *Any known allergies* that make the breathing worse? Discussed in the answer to question 10 and below.

● *Past history* of asthma, eczema or hay fever? Discussed in the answer to question 10.

● *Family history* of asthma, eczema or hay fever? Discussed in the answer to question 10.

Notes about the questions

Time of day. Like left ventricular failure, asthma often wakes patients in the middle of the night, although whereas the nocturnal dyspnoea associated with heart failure is due to congestion of the lungs, in asthma it is probably due to exaggeration of the diurnal narrowing of the airways that occurs normally at night. In much the same way, breathlessness on rising in the morning is probably due in part to the same mechanism and also to the effects of any mucus collecting overnight.

Allergic asthma. As discussed in the answer to question 10 this may be precipitated by pollen, animal dander (minute particles of fur and feathers), or for example by mite particles in house dust. Seasonal asthma may be worse when the pollen or mould count is high. Asthma in the spring is usually associated with flower pollen, in the summer with grass pollen and in the autumn with moulds.

ii   *Bronchitis*

● *The colour of the sputum?* Unless infected, generally it is white; however with infection it usually becomes yellow or green (see page 253).

● *Do you, or have you ever smoked?* If so, how many per day, for how many years?

● *Time of year, seasonal variation?* Generally the breathlessness of chronic obstructive airways disease tends to be worse in the winter. Acute infective exacerbations also tend to occur in the winter.

● *Time of day?* Perhaps because of overnight mucus collection, like asthma, the breathlessness of chronic obstructive airways disease tends to be worse on rising in the morning. However, although it may be associated with breathlessness on lying flat, it is unusual for chronic obstructive airways disease to cause nocturnal dyspnoea.

Signs and investigation
Questions

13i   List the specific investigations you should order in *an outpatient* suspected of having asthma. How are peak expiratory flow rate measurements and measurement of FEV₁/VC used in the diagnosis and assessment of the response to therapy?

ii   What are prick skin tests? What is the place of prick skin tests in the modern assessment of asthma, and what is the place of desensitisation in the treatment of asthma?

14i   List the specific features of the examination that must be checked for and recorded in severe life threatening asthma.

ii   List the specific investigations that should be ordered for such a patient when admitted to hospital.

Answers

13   Outpatient investigations; prick skin tests

i   The specific investigations of an outpatient suspected of having asthma are:

●   *Full blood count.* This may show an eosinophilia in both extrinsic and intrinsic asthma.

●   *Lung function tests.* The hallmark of asthma is variability of airways obstruction. This can be confirmed by asking the patient to record their peak expiratory flow rate three or four times per day over a period of several days or a week or so. Marked variability, particularly with depressed readings on rising in the morning (the so-called *morning dip*), supports a diagnosis of asthma.

The response to treatment can be monitored by making recordings before and after treatment. Improvement of more than 15–20% after inhalation of a ß₂ adrenergic agonist is generally taken to be associated with asthma.

The response to a therapeutic trial of oral steroids should be monitored by recording the peak expiratory flow rate several times per day over a period of two weeks or so.

Measurements of FEV₁ and VC should be made at each clinic visit.

●   *Chest x-ray.* As it is usually normal, routine x-ray of the chest may be unnecessary in otherwise well young outpatients.

ii   *Prick tests* involve the injection of minute amounts of allergen into the epidermis and observation of whether or not there is a wheal and flare reaction. Because the tests are positive in about 20% of persons without any clinical evidence of allergic disease, and because the results of the tests correlate poorly with clinical events and only very occasionally lead to any alteration of management, they are only rarely indicated in normal clinical practice. Such an instance might be where a single antigen, such as an antigen encountered at work, is suspected of causing asthma.

Similarly, because it may cause anaphylaxis, desensitisation, in which the patient is given regular intramuscular injections of increasing amounts of antigen, is dangerous and has no place in the treatment of most cases of asthma. The only situation in which it might be indicated is where a patient has been demonstrated to be allergic to a single allergen and symptoms are disabling.

14   Severe life threatening asthma

i   The specific features of the examination that must be checked for and recorded in severe life threatening asthma are:

● *The severity of breathlessness.* The attack is serious if the patient is breathless at rest or is unable to speak properly.

● *The presence of cyanosis.* As it may reflect respiratory failure, the presence of any cyanosis has serious implications.

● *The use of accessory muscles.* This sign reflects serious airways obstruction causing increased work of breathing and carries the implication that the patient may become dangerously fatigued.

● *Auscultation.* During an attack of asthma the breath sounds usually consist of a growling wheeze with prolonged expiration. However, with extreme airways obstruction the chest may become silent, hence the term 'beware the silent chest'.

● *Clinical measurements.* Severe asthma is suggested by:
Respiratory rate: > 30 breaths per minute
Pulse rate: > 110 beats per minute
Pulsus paradoxus: > 10 mmHg
Peak expiratory flow rate: < 100 litres per minute
The pathophysiology and simplest way of measuring pulsus paradoxus is discussed on page 147. Serial readings of peak expiratory flow rate are required to monitor the patient's progress.

ii   The specific investigations of a case of severe life threatening asthma are:

● *Chest x-ray.* Although it is usually normal or shows only hyperinflation and is therefore of debatable value, the main justification for asking for a chest x-ray in severe asthma is to exclude a pneumothorax needing urgent drainage. Occasionally the x-ray may also show consolidation due to pneumonia or help differentiate bronchial from cardiac asthma, or more rarely show the transient or flitting shadows associated with aspergillosis.

● *Blood gases.* Mild asthma is associated with hyperventilation causing $PaCO_2$ to fall. A severe attack is signalled by a normal or rising $PaCO_2$. Serial observations must be made to monitor progress in such a case.

● *Urea and electrolytes.* The respiratory alkalosis caused by the hyperventilation associated with asthma may result in *hypokalaemia* that in turn may be associated with *cardiac arrhythmias*. The explanation of such hypokalaemia is that in the presence of a respiratory alkalosis the kidney reduces its production of HCO_3^- ions for distribution to the circulation and H^+ ions for excretion in the distal renal tubule. As a consequence of the reduced production of H^+ ions, K^+ ions rather than H^+ ions are exchanged for Na⁺ ions in the distal tubule. The result is an increased loss of potassium in the urine and hypokalaemia in the blood.

● *Electrocardiogram.* Usually the least necessary investigation. However, occasionally it may show ST depression due to strain in the leads that reflect events in the right ventricle, that is in the inferior leads II, III and aVf, and the chest leads over the right ventricle, namely leads V_1 and V_2.

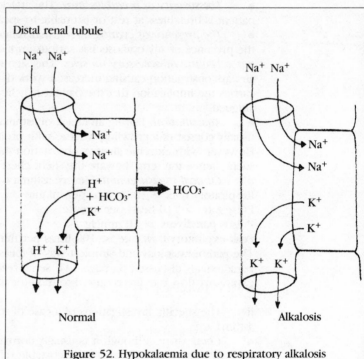

Figure 52. Hypokalaemia due to respiratory alkalosis

Outpatient treatment

Questions

15 What are the aims of the treatment of asthma? By what means are they achieved?

16 List the five different types of drugs available for the treatment of asthma. What are their modes of action? In what forms may they be given? Comment on any limitations to their use.

17 The treatment of outpatients with asthma is tailored to suit the severity of the condition. Suggest a strategy giving the order and form in which the five groups of drugs listed above should be prescribed for:

i   *Occasional* wheeze or breathlessness.

ii   *Regular* wheeze or breathlessness.

iii   Chronic disabling asthma.

Answers

15   The aims of the treatment of asthma

These are quite simply the restoration and maintenance of open airways. This is achieved by:

● *Drugs.* Although drugs are the main means of keeping the airways open, hypnotherapy and acupuncture help some patients, whilst the following factors are also very important:

● *Reassurance.* Most experienced clinicians know of asthmatic patients who have improved with reassurance alone. Reassurance seems to allay the anxiety and fear that accompanies breathlessness, and also possibly helps resolve stresses acting as a trigger to the asthma.

● *Avoidance of precipitating factors.* General measures such as changing from feather pillows, not having a carpet in the bedroom and avoiding individual animals known to precipitate attacks help some patients. In addition, the likelihood of exercise induced asthma may be reduced by prophylactic inhalation of a $ß_2$ adrenergic agonist or cromoglycate before exercise. On the other hand, obsessive attempts to avoid widespread allergens by manoeuvres such as hoovering away all house dust are usually unsuccessful.

16   The five types of drug used in the treatment of asthma, their modes of action, forms of delivery and limitations of use

● $ß_2$ adrenergic agonists
● Methylxanthines
● Corticosteroids
● Cromoglycate
● Parasympathetic antagonists

$ß_2$ adrenergic agonists

As indicated on page 228 the $ß_2$ adrenergic agonists mimic the $ß_2$ and to a slight extent the $ß_1$ actions of adrenaline. Therapeutically their main action is to cause relaxation of bronchial smooth muscle and stabilisation of mast cells. Within the cell they are thought to activate the enzyme adenyl cyclase leading to an increase of cAMP.

The $ß_2$ adrenergic agonists are used in the treatment of asthma and those cases of chronic obstructive airways disease in which there is a reversible component. Salbutamol is the most commonly prescribed preparation. Although available orally as a tablet, slow release capsule or elixir, for routine use the most effective way of administering salbutamol is as a pressurised aerosol. For emergency use it is as effective as a nebulised aerosol delivered from a nebuliser as by intravenous infusion, and less likely to cause side effects. The preferred ways of administering salbutamol, and the other $ß_2$ adrenergic agonists that are available in such forms, are therefore as a pressurised aerosol or via a nebuliser. However, if they are prescribed as an aerosol it is important to ensure that the patient knows how to administer them, as surveys have shown that up to 30% fail to do so correctly.

Side effects. At recommended dosages side effects are unusual and consist of palpitations due to stimulation of ß1 adrenoreceptors in the heart, and tremors of voluntary muscles due to stimulation of ß2 adrenoreceptors on muscle fibres.

Apart from salbutamol, the other most commonly used ß2 adrenergic agonists are terbutaline, fenoterol and rimiterol.

Methylxanthines

Aminophylline and theophylline are the most commonly prescribed examples of this group of drugs whose action is to relax bronchial smooth muscle and prevent the activation of mast cells by an as yet unknown mechanism.

The methylxanthines tend to be second line drugs because (a) they frequently cause nausea and dyspepsia, and (b) their therapeutic and toxic blood levels are nearly the same, that is they have a narrow *therapeutic index*.

However, they may help those in whom inhaled broncho-dilators do not effect full bronchodilation, and because they are fairly long acting, taken before bed they may relieve cough, wheeze or breathlessness in some patients at night.

The mode of administration of the xanthines is as a tablet, intravenous infusion or injection, or as a suppository. Because it may cause vascular collapse, intravenous aminophylline should be given slowly at a rate of no more than 50 mg per minute to a maximum of 250–500 mg, stopping if the patient feels unwell. Caution is also needed when giving these drugs intravenously to patients who have already received them orally within the previous 12 hours. In general, in this situation the dose should be halved.

Corticosteroids

These drugs are thought to have several actions in asthma:
●   Inhibition of the enzyme phospholipase in the wall of the mast cell. As explained on page 233, this results in reduced production of arachidonic acid which in turn results in reduced production of bronchoconstrictor leukotrienes and prostaglandins. Interruption of phospholipid metabolism may also result in reduced production of platelet activating factor (PAF), discussed on page 232.
●   It is thought that corticosteroids also reduce the activity of mast cells by stabilising lysozyme enzymes within the cell.
●   In addition steroids also enhance the relaxing effect of ß2 adrenergic agonists on bronchial smooth muscle.

Steroids are administered by inhaler, tablet or by intramuscular or intravenous injection. By injection they take about 8 hours to have an effect. By inhalation an effect may not be discernible for 2 or 3 weeks, which means that by inhalation they should be used as prophylactics against future events and not for acute attacks. The advantage of inhaled steroids is that as they are delivered directly to their site of action, recommended doses of less than 1 mg per day have the same effect as prednisolone 7½ mg daily taken by tablet.

The use of systemic steroids is limited by their side effects. These include the development of truncal and facial obesity, hypertension, diabetes, psychosis, and catabolism of protein resulting in osteoporosis, thinning of the skin and loss of muscle bulk.

Cromoglycate

Initially this drug was thought to act by stabilising the membrane of the mast cell. Recently, however, this has been doubted although it is still thought that part of its action is due to inhibition of the release of humoral mediators. Cromoglycate is inhaled and because it takes up to 2 or 3 weeks to be effective is a prophylactic against future events and has no place in the treatment of acute attacks. Relatively few patients are helped by it. These tend to be children with extrinsic asthma, although occasional patients with intrinsic asthma may be helped by it. Cromoglycate has no important side effects.

Parasympathetic antagonists

These drugs are less effective bronchodilators than the ß2 adrenergic agonists and are used mainly in the treatment of partially reversible chronic obstructive airways disease, although they may also help some patients with asthma. They act by competitively inhibiting, that is blocking the receptor sites for bronchoconstrictor acetylcholine released by the vagus nerve to the lung. Because it causes systemic effects and a dry mouth, atropine is not suitable for inhalation. However, ipratropium acts more specifically on the airways and may be administered by either pressurised aerosol or nebuliser, usually in conjunction with a ß2 adrenergic agonist.

17   A plan based upon the severity of the disease for giving each of the five medications in the outpatient treatment of asthma

The following plan is simple and provides a step-wise scheme based upon the severity of the condition:

i   *Occasional wheezing or breathlessness*
●   A ß2 adrenergic agonist by pressurised aerosol, to be used as required.

ii   *Regular wheezing or breathlessness*
●   A ß2 adrenergic agonist by pressurised aerosol, regularly

three to four times per day,

+

Either
● A steroid pressurised aerosol, regularly as prophylaxis,
or
● Cromoglycate inhaled regularly as prophylaxis for those few
patients who respond to it.

If these measures are not sufficient, inhaled ipratropium or tablets
of a methylxanthine may be added.

iii   *Chronic disabling asthma*
In addition to the above medications:
● The first move here should be a trial of a ß2 adrenergic
agonist ± ipratropium by *nebuliser* up to four times per day,
rather than by pressurised aerosol.
● The above medications plus the smallest necessary
maintenance dose of oral steroids, for example prednisolone 5-10
mg each morning.

Hospital treatment
Questions

18   List in detail the *hospital* treatment of a severely breathless
asthmatic patient.
19   What are the indications for artificial ventilation in such
patients?

Answers

**18   The hospital treatment of a severely breathless
asthmatic patient**

Because deaths from asthma continue to occur all severely
breathless asthmatic patients should be admitted to hospital as a
matter of urgency and should receive the following treatment:
● *Reassurance*. The value of this has already been discussed in
the answer to question 15.
● *Oxygen*. As there is no danger of suppressing anoxic drive,
asthmatics may be given oxygen in high concentrations, for
instance via an MC mask.
● *Bronchodilators*. A nebulised ß2 adrenergic agonist together
with nebulised ipratropium should be given on admission and
every 4 hours until the patient is better when the drugs may be
administered by ordinary aerosol.
● *Steroids*. All asthmatics ill enough to warrant admission to
hospital should receive systemic corticosteroids. On the first day
intravenous hydrocortisone 100 mg three times per day should be
given. Thereafter an oral preparation such as prednisolone 40 mg
each morning should be given for 14 days, followed by either
stopping the drug, or maintaining the patient on a steroid inhaler,
or a steroid inhaler together with the smallest amount of oral

corticosteroid necessary to keep the condition under control.
* *Aminophylline.* Usually it is sufficient to give the nebulised bronchodilators mentioned above. However, in very severe cases these may be augmented by intravenous or infused aminophylline along the lines suggested in the answer to question 16.
* *Physiotherapy.* So long as it is gentle and does not exhaust the patient, physiotherapy may help expectoration and clearing of the airways.
NOTES:
* *Antibiotics.* It should be remembered that the sputum of an asthmatic may be discoloured by either infection or eosinophils. Unless the sputum is discoloured by infection, antibiotics are not usually required.
* *Sedation.* Patients have died after receiving as little as diazepam 5 mg. Although it may be tempting to consider relieving a patient's anxiety, sedation should never be given.

19 The indications for artificial ventilation in severe asthma

Artificial ventilation, usually for 24-48 hours, is indicated for:
* Developing respiratory failure indicated by a rising of $PaCO_2$, above about 7.0 kPa.
* Exhaustion.

Further Reading

Crofton J, Douglas A (1981). *Respiratory Disease*, 3rd edition. Blackwell Scientific Publications, Oxford. Chapter 28, bronchial asthma.
Weatherall DJ, Ledingham JGG, Warrell DA (eds) (1987). *Oxford Textbook of Medicine*, 2nd edition. Oxford University Press, Oxford. Asthma, pp 15.75-82.

Chapter 17
Chronic Obstructive
Airways Disease
(COAD)

Chronic bronchitis and emphysema (also known as chronic airways limitation).

Definitions; causative factors
Questions

1   Define the terms 'chronic bronchitis' and 'emphysema'.
2   List and briefly discusss the main causative factors, such as smoking, associated with the development of COAD. Include a note about alpha₁, anti-trypsin deficiency and the development of COAD.

Answers

1   Definitions

● *Chronic bronchitis* is defined as a chronic cough productive of sputum for 3 months or more during 2 or more consecutive years, conditions such as bronchiectasis and tuberculosis having been excluded.
● *Emphysema* is defined as an increase in the size of the air spaces distal to the terminal bronchioles and is associated with destruction of alveolar walls. The destruction also involves the capillaries that run over the alveoli and the supporting elastin fibres. Both total lung capacity (the volume of the lungs at the top of inspiration) and residual volume (the volume of the lungs at the end of forced expiration) are abnormally large in patients with emphysema, although it should be noted that emphysema is not just overdistension of air spaces of the type seen in asthma.

Note that chronic bronchitis is defined in clinical terms and emphysema in pathological terms, and that in most patients with chronic obstructive airways disease, as discussed on page 229, there is a mixture of the two conditions.

2   The main causative factors associated with the development of COAD

These may be divided into:
● *Environmental factors* about which a great deal is known.

• *Intrinsic or constitutional factors* within the patient about which little is known.

Environmental factors

• *Smoking*. Almost all patients with clinically significant COAD are or have been regular smokers. The mortality of COAD is linearly related to the number of cigarettes smoked. Experimental studies of smoking in animals have produced histological changes of both chronic bronchitis and emphysema.

• *Air pollution*. This is less important than smoking in the causation of COAD, but nonetheless the incidence of the disease is greater among people living in cities than in the country, although the difference has decreased with the control of air pollution. The pollutants in the atmosphere that are responsible are mainly sulphuric acid and particulate matter.

• *Sex*. Due mainly to smoking, the incidence of COAD is greater among males than females.

• *Social class*. The incidence of COAD is smaller among people with a professional occupation than among manual workers. The difference cannot be wholly explained by differences in the smoking habits of the two groups, and may be related in part to housing, and the fact that frequent respiratory tract infections in childhood are commoner among the poor and are possibly a factor in the development of COAD in adulthood.

• *Occupation*. The incidence of COAD is greater among persons exposed to organic and inorganic dusts, such as miners.

Intrinsic factors

• Intrinsic predisposing factors are suggested by the fact that only about 15% of heavy smokers develop clinically significant COAD.

• alpha$_1$ *anti-trypsin deficiency*. The serum enzyme alpha$_1$ anti-trypsin is an anti-protease whose role is possibly to protect tissues from autodigestion by proteases in the blood. Low levels of the enzymes are associated with raised amounts of the enzymes, elastase and collagenase, in the blood, and the development of cirrhosis in childhood or emphysema by early middle age. The condition should therefore be suspected in anyone developing emphysema before age 45 years.

The condition is subject to Mendelian inheritance. In normals the serum level of alpha$_1$ anti-trypsin is > 250 mg%. In homozygotes the serum level is > 50 mg%, and in heterozygotes 50–250 mg%.

Pathology (i)
Questions

3i   What are the main structural differences between bronchi and bronchioles?

ii   In what part of the bronchial tree does most resistance to

the flow of air occur firstly in normals, and secondly in COAD?
4i   Describe the main histological changes in both the large and small airways in chronic bronchitis.
ii   What cells are thought to be responsible for the destruction of lung tissue in emphysema?
5   What is an acinus of the lung? Name and briefly describe the two main histological types of emphysema.

Answers

3i   The main structural differences between bronchi and bronchioles

Bronchi contain compound mucous glands that extend into the submucosa, and also supporting cartilage within their walls. Bronchioles contain neither, although the mucosa of a bronchiole does contain individual mucus producing goblet cells.

3ii   The anatomical sites of resistance to flow of air

●   *In normals* the main site of resistance to the flow of air is the trachea and bronchi. This is because the total cross-sectional area of the small airways is so great that any resistance to the flow of air in this part of the lungs is minimal.
●   *In COAD* the main site of resistance to the flow of air is the small airways. This is because of narrowing, distortion and collapse of small bronchi and bronchioles.

4i   The main histological changes in the large and small airways in chronic bronchitis

●   *In the trachea and larger bronchi* the main changes associated with chronic bronchitis are an increase in the number and size of the submucosal compound mucous glands. Smooth muscle hyperplasia also occurs, although its significance is not clear.
●   *In the smaller bronchi and bronchioles* the characteristic changes of chronic bronchitis are an increase in the number of individual goblet mucus producing cells within the mucosa and an inflammatory infiltrate consisting mainly of neutrophils and macrophages that release proteolytic enzymes and toxic oxidising substances that cause fibrosis, narrowing and distortion of the airways.

4ii   The cellular changes associated with the destructive lesion of emphysema

Macrophages and to a lesser extent neutrophils accumulate in the lung and die, releasing proteolytic enzymes such as elastase that digest the walls of the alveoli, the capillaries running over them, and the supporting elastin fibres.

5   The acinus and the two main histological types of emphysema

The acinus of the lung is the gas exchange unit, that is the respiratory bronchiole together with the several alveoli it serves.

The two main types of emphysema are:
- *Central acinar emphysema* involving mainly the respiratory bronchiole.
- *Pan-acinar emphysema* involving the whole acinus.

In severe cases, both types of emphysema may be found.

Pathology (ii)
Questions

6   Describe, and if helpful, draw a simple diagram showing why loss of elastic recoil is important in emphysema.

7   List the mechanisms, such as abnormalities of ventilation/perfusion, that contribute to the breathlessness of patients with emphysema.

Answers

6   The importance of the loss of elastic recoil in emphysema

Fibres of elastin act as supporting strands between small airways and alveoli. As illustrated, a simple way to think of elastin is as lines or stays holding up a tent.

During inspiration the negative pressure created within the thorax causes the airways and alveoli to distend and air to rush in. This is associated with stretching of the elastin fibres.

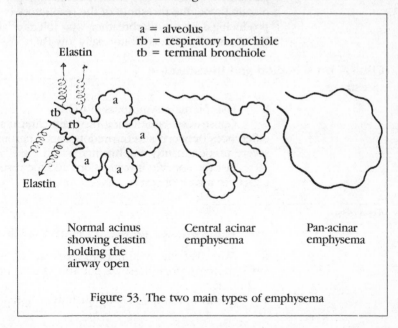

a = alveolus
rb = respiratory bronchiole
tb = terminal bronchiole

Elastin

tb
rb

a
a
a
a

Elastin

Normal acinus showing elastin holding the airway open

Central acinar emphysema

Pan-acinar emphysema

Figure 53. The two main types of emphysema

During expiration the energy stored in these stretched fibres provides a force known as *elastic recoil* that tends to collapse the lung and helps to empty the alveoli. At the same time other fibres of elastin provide radial traction to the small airways, holding them open and preventing their closure under the influence of the crushing pressure created by the force of expiration.

In emphysema elastin is largely destroyed. From what has been said above it follows that (a) elastic recoil and the help it provides to emptying the lung is largely lost, and (b) without elastin to hold them open, small airways tend to collapse and close under the force of expiration, causing trapping of air within the alveoli.

7 The mechanisms contributing to the breathlessness of patients with emphysema

- *Increase of airways resistance* due to narrowing of the airways and loss of elastic recoil. This results in increased respiratory effort and an increase in the energy and work of breathing.
- *Impaired diffusion of gases* as a result of destruction of the alveolar/capillary gas exchange surfaces.
- *Mismatching of ventilation and perfusion of the lung* as a result of airways obstruction causing impaired ventilation and destruction of capillaries causing impaired perfusion.
- *Resetting of the sensitivity of the respiratory centre*. The threshold of the respiratory centre to stimulation by carbon dioxide and hydrogen ions is lowered in the pink puffer emphysematous type of patient and results in breathlessness and faster than normal breathing with maintenance of normal blood gases. By contrast, in the chronic bronchitic patient of the blue bloating type, the threshold of the respiratory centre is raised, producing a 'lazy' underbreather who tolerates an abnormally high $PaCO_2$, usually with an abnormally low PaO_2.

Clinical presentation and investigation
Questions

8 List the main symptoms of COAD.
9 Construct a table listing the main clinical and investigative differences between severe predominantly chronic bronchitis and severe predominantly emphysema.
10 List the specific investigations and the results you might expect in a case of severe mixed COAD.

Answers

8 The main symptoms of COAD

- *None*. Patients with mild to moderate COAD often have very few symptoms. Breathlessness due to COAD is unusual until FEV_1 < 2 litres.
- *Sputum production*. The quantity of sputum produced is of

little help in assessing the severity of disease. By definition, in patients at the bronchitic end of the spectrum the production of sputum is an early feature. On the other hand at the emphysematous end of the spectrum sputum production is usually scanty.

Any sputum produced is usually white, but during infective exacerbations generally turns green or yellow.

●   *Breathlessness.* This is mainly on exertion, is associated with $FEV_1 < 2$ litres per second, and possibly due to the accumulation of overnight secretions, tends to be worse on rising in the morning. Many patients with COAD suffer with orthopnoea and sleep in a relatively upright position.

●   *Swelling of the ankles and legs.* This is evidence of developing *cor pulmonale*, the term used to describe right sided heart failure secondary to lung disease of any cause.

●   *Drowsiness, confusion and agitation.* These symptoms occur with carbon dioxide retention and narcosis.

9   Table listing the main clinical and investigative differences between severe predominantly chronic bronchitis and severe predominantly emphysema

Answer on page 254.

10   The specific investigations and likely results in severe COAD

●   *Full blood count.* As implied on page 254, this might reveal polycythaemia.

●   *Sputum culture.* The organisms involved in exacerbations are usually *Streptococcus pneumoniae* or *Haemophilus influenzae*. Because of this, routine sputum culture is not required, except for patients who fail to respond to a course of a broad spectrum antibiotic.

●   *Chest x-ray.* In addition to the changes described in the answer to question 9, chest x-ray may also show consolidation due to pneumonia or changes due to a carcinoma (discussed on page 285.

●   *Lung function tests.* These tests are mandatory, and patients with COAD are incompletely documented until FEV_1 and VC have been measured to assess the severity of the disease. Interpretation of the results is discussed on pages 222–223.

Because it is more conveniently measured, peak expiratory flow rate may be recorded where repeated measurements are required to assess progress over a period of hours or days.

●   *Blood gases.* Serial measurements to monitor progress and responses to therapy are required in acutely ill patients with respiratory failure.

Table listing the main clinical and investigative differences between severe predominantly chronic bronchitis and severe predominantly emphysema

Clinical feature	Severe chronic bronchitis	Severe emphysema
Sputum	Copious	Scanty
Breathlessness	Not particularly breathless. Lazy underbreather	Breathless on least effort. Overbreather
General appearance	Cyanosed blue bloater. Build normal or overweight	Pink puffer. Usually thin
Chest	Of normal appearance	Barrel chest; ribs horizontal
Breath sounds	Reduced with prolonged expiration	Reduced with prolonged expiration
Cor pulmonale	Typically occurs with infective exacerbations	Unusual, except as a terminal event
Investigations:		
Chest x-ray	Typically shows only increased bronchovascular marking of the lung fields*	Typically shows: Long chest Flat diaphragm Increased sternocardiac space. Due to destruction, reduced bronchovascular markings
Blood gases	PaO_2 often low $PaCO_2$ often high	PaO_2 usually normal $PaCO_2$ usually normal
Polycythaemia	Occasional	Rare
Lung compliance (ease with which the lung is inflated)	Normal	Increased (due to loss of elastic recoil the lung is easily inflated)
Diffusing capacity	Normal	Reduced due to destruction of lung tissue
Pulmonary hypertension (constriction of the pulmonary arteries due to anoxia)	Common, worsening with exercise	Uncommon, sometimes occurring with exercise

* It is important to appreciate that even in patients who are dying of the condition, the chest x-ray in chronic bronchitis may appear normal except for a little increase in the marking of the lung fields.

Outpatient treatment
Questions

11   What is the main aim of the treatment of COAD?
12   Considering patients outside hospital, describe the maintenance treatment you would prescribe or at least try in patients with breathlessness due to COAD. How would you monitor the response?
13   What are the indications for domiciliary oxygen in such patients?

Answers

11   The main aim of the treatment of COAD

●   The main aim of the treatment of COAD is to restore oxygenation of the tissues as a result of
a   Removal of secretions.
b   Effecting bronchodilation if possible.
However, usually the disease is less reversible than asthma.
●   A further aim is to prevent smoking. Stopping halves the annual rate of deterioration of FEV_1 to about 40 ml, compared with about 80 ml in those who continue to smoke.

12   Outpatient maintenance treatment of patients with COAD

●   *Introduction*. Although many patients with COAD have irreversible or only partially reversible airways obstruction every breathless patient with the condition should be assessed to effect all possible bronchodilation.
●   *Monitoring the response to therapy*. This is done by monitoring both the patient's subjective response to therapy, and by measuring changes in FEV_1 or peak expiratory flow rate together with the distance the patient is able to walk in, say, 6 or 12 minutes before and after therapy. Only those drugs that have been clearly shown to help should be prescribed.
●   *Bronchodilators*. With the exception of cromoglycate, which has no place in the treatment of COAD, the drugs used to obtain maximal bronchodilatation are largely the same as those discussed on page 243 for the treatment of asthma.
●   *Steroids*. Up to about 25% of patients respond to regular steroid inhalation or a small maintenance dose of oral steroids. In order to seek out a clinically useful reversible component to their disability all patients with severe COAD should have a therapeutic trial of oral steroids, for instance, prednisolone 40 mg each morning for 2 weeks.
●   *Antibiotics*. Infective exacerbations signalled by increased breathlessness and purulent sputum infected with either *Streptococcus pneumoniae* or *Haemophilus influenzae* usually respond to a 5 day course of a broad spectrum oral antibiotic such as ampicillin, tetracycline, trimethoprim or a cephalosporin.

- *Mucolytics.* These drugs are rarely helpful.
- *Regular exercise.* Although it does not improve lung function, exercise training usually increases exercise tolerance by more than 10%, probably partly by a training effect on the muscles, but mainly from an increased sense of wellbeing.
- *Domiciliary oxygen.* See below.

13 The indications for domiciliary oxygen in patients with severe COAD

- Domiciliary oxygen is indicated in patients who are breathless during their terminal illness.
- In addition domiciliary oxygen may be used to improve the prognosis of a small group of patients with severe COAD. These are patients in *stable* respiratory failure, PaO_2 persistently < 7.3 kPa (55 mmHg) and $FEV_1 < 1.5$ litres/second. The oxygen is administered by nasal catheter at a rate of 2 litres per minute or at a rate sufficient to raise PaO_2 to 8 kPa (60 mmHg) for not less than 15 hours per day (including sleeping). Given in this way the number of patients surviving 3–5 years is increased by 20%.
- As a general rule oxygen is not indicated for breathlessness without hypoxaemia.

Hospital treatment
Questions

14i Define the term 'respiratory failure'. Briefly describe the two accepted types of respiratory failure.

ii Describe the treatment you would prescribe for an ill drowsy cyanosed patient admitted to hospital with respiratory failure due to COAD.

15 What are the indications for artificial ventilation of such patients? What reservations would you have about ventilating such a patient? What practical guide can be used to decide whether the patient is terminal or whether ventilation is justified?

Answers

14i Definition of the term respiratory failure, and the two accepted types of respiratory failure

Respiratory failure is defined as impaired gas exchange in the lungs, and is associated with deranged blood gases. The degree of derangement required for the definition is somewhat arbitrary, but is generally accepted as $PaO_2 < 8$ kPa (approximately 60 mmHg) and/or $PaCO_2 > 7$ kPa (approximately 50 mmHg).

Two types of respiratory failure are recognised:

- *Type I respiratory failure.* In this condition *ventilation is adequate enabling CO_2 to be blown off, but oxygenation of the blood is impaired* resulting in a low PaO_2 and a $PaCO_2$ which is either normal or low. Examples of this type of respiratory failure are breathlessness and hypoxaemia due to pulmonary fibrosis, left ventricular failure and conditions in which there is marked mismatching of ventilation and perfusion such as pulmonary embolus and pneumonia.

• *Type II respiratory failure*. In this condition *ventilation is inadequate* resulting in a raised $PaCO_2$ as well as a low PaO_2. Examples of this are conditions such as weakness of the respiratory muscles due to polyneuropathy, or severe life threatening asthma, or underbreathing as a result of impaired sensitivity of the respiratory centre in COAD of the bronchitic blue bloating type.

14ii Treatment of an ill drowsy cyanosed patient with respiratory failure due to COAD

The principles by which oxygenation of the tissues is increased are discussed in detail below and include:
• Adequate ventilation of the lungs and clearance of secretions.
• Administration of oxygen in a controlled manner.
• Bronchodilation.
• Administration of a broad spectrum antibiotic to treat the infection that is usually present.
• Other measures that include the use of corticosteroids, diuretics, respiratory stimulants and the avoidance of sedatives.

• *Adequate ventilaton and removal of secretions*.
Physiotherapy is one of the most important aspects of the management of patients with respiratory failure due to COAD, firstly to effect expectoration of secretions, and secondly to encourage the patient to breathe and blow off carbon dioxide and take in oxygen. To this end drowsy patients should be visited every hour by a nurse, doctor or physiotherapist specifically to encourage coughing and deep breathing.
• *Oxygen*. Patients with respiratory failure due to COAD are usually at the lazy breather end of the spectrum and tolerate a chronically raised $PaCO_2$, relying on anoxia for respiratory drive. The administration of high concentrations of oxygen can suppress this drive and cause dangerous respiratory depression. Caution is therefore needed when giving oxygen, the aim being to increase tissue oxygenation without depressing ventilation. This is achieved by giving oxygen at strictly controlled concentrations. Masks are used that work on the Venturi effect, delivering oxygen in fixed concentrations of 24%, 28% or 32% (air containing 21%). Initially 24% oxygen is given and the patient's clinical response monitored after ½–1 hour for signs of increased respiratory depression, and if necessary, blood gases measured for evidence of deterioration. If 24% oxygen is well tolerated, 28% may be tried cautiously, monitoring the patient as before.
• *Bronchodilators*. A $ß_2$ adrenergic agonist together with the parasympathetic antagonist, ipratropium, should be administered by nebuliser to every patient who is ill with respiratory failure due

to COAD. A methylxanthine may also be given. The actions and administration of these drugs are discussed on pages 243–245.

● *Antibiotics*. As previously stated, 90% of exacerbations of COAD are associated with infection due to *Streptococcus pneumoniae* or *Haemophilus influenzae*, both of which usually respond to a 5 day course of a broad spectrum antibiotic such as ampicillin, tetracycline, trimethoprim or a cephalosporin.

● *Corticosteroids*. Opinion is divided about the need for steroids in these patients, although it is generally accepted that they should be given if bronchospasm is suspected. In the author's opinion, in practice this means giving a steroid, for instance oral prednisolone 20 mg each morning for about a week.

● *Diuretics*. A loop diuretic or a thiazide should be given for oedema or more severe right sided heart failure, together if necessary with a potassium retaining diuretic. A detailed account of diuretic therapy is given on page 44.

● *Respiratory stimulants*. Patients failing to respond to the above medications and making insufficient respiratory effort may be given a cautious trial infusion of the respiratory stimulant, doxapram, a watch being kept for side effects such as tremor, agitation, tachycardia and convulsions.

● *Sedation*. Sedatives may increase respiratory depression in patients who are ill with COAD and therefore should never be given. Deaths have occurred in such patients following the administration of just one sleeping pill.

15   The indications for and reservations about artificial ventilation in patients who are drowsy with respiratory failure due to COAD

● *Indications*. Artificial ventilation is indicated in such a patient who is deteriorating despite the measures discussed in the previous answer, and in whom there is evidence of increasing carbon dioxide narcosis suggested by increasing drowsiness, confusion or agitation, decreased respiratory effort and a $PaCO_2$ rising to 10 kPa (75 mmHg) or more.

● *Selection of patients*. It is important to appreciate that only patients who are likely to get off the respirator should be ventilated, and that it is unkind and a disservice to both the patient and their family to ventilate those who are truly terminal. Whilst no rule covers every contingency, in most instances a good working guide is to consider the patient's previous level of activity. If they were able to go out of their home before the present exacerbation it will probably be possible to wean them off the ventilator. Those with irreversible disease who have been confined to bed or their room for weeks before admission should probably not be ventilated.

Further Reading

Crofton J, Douglas A (1981). *Respiratory Diseases*, 3rd edition. Blackwell Scientific Publications, Oxford. Chapter 20, chronic bronchitis and emphysema.

Weatherall DJ, Ledingham JGG, Warrell DA (eds) (1987). *Oxford Textbook of Medicine*, 2nd edition. Oxford University Press, Oxford. Chronic bronchitis, emphysema and chronic obstructive airway disease, pp 15.83–91.

Chapter 18
Interstitial Lung Disease (ILD)

Also known as alveolitis, and often loosely referred to as pulmonary fibrosis

Definition; classification; mechanical effects

Questions

1   Define the term 'interstitial lung disease'.
2   Give a classification of the various types of ILD, listing two or three examples in each group.
3   What are the three main ways in which ILD affects the mechanics of the lung?

Answers

1   Definition

The interstitial lung diseases are defined as a group of non-infectious, non-malignant inflammatory disorders of the lower respiratory tract associated with an inflammatory infiltrate, damage of the alveolar wall and thickening of the interstitium between the alveoli, usually with fibrosis.

2   Classification with examples of the various types of ILD

More than 180 forms of ILD have been described. The most useful classification is based upon the aetiology of the condition.

Cause unknown	Inhaled inorganic dust	Inhaled organic dust	Drugs
● Sarcoidosis	● Coal miner's pneumoconiosis	Extrinsic allergic alveolitis	● Nitrofurantoin ● Amiodarone
● Cryptogenic fibrosing alveolitis	● Silicosis	● Farmer's lung	● Anti-cancer drugs:
● Fibrosing alveolitis associated with the collagenoses	● Asbestosis	● Bird fancier's lung ● Mushroom worker's lung	Methotrexate Cyclophosphamide Bleomycin Melphalan Busulphan
● Goodpasture's syndrome		● Maltworker's lung	
● Wegener's granulomatosis		—	

In farmer's lung, mushroom worker's lung and maltworker's lung the organic dust is the spore of various fungi. In bird fancier's lung the sensitising particles are a plasma protein passed in the stools of the bird.

3 The three main ways ILD affects the mechanics of the lung

● *Increased work of breathing.* Due mainly to the patient breathing harder because the lungs are stiff and less compliant than normal.
● *Mismatching of ventilation and perfusion.* As mentioned in a previous section, these two aspects of lung function are normally matched in such a way as to ensure optimum exchange of oxygen and carbon dioxide between the alveoli and capillaries. Although the main cause of reduced transfer of gases in ILD is often thought to be damage and thickening of the alveolar wall, in fact it is due mainly to mismatching of ventilation and perfusion.
● *Impaired diffusion of gases across the damaged, thickened alveolar wall.* As stated above this is a smaller factor in the impaired exchange of gases in ILD than abnormalities of ventilation and perfusion.

Definition of sarcoidosis and pneumoconiosis, and associations
Questions

4i Define the term 'sarcoidosis'.
 ii Define the term 'pneumoconiosis'.
 iii With which occupations are the commoner pneumoconioses associated?
 iv What is Caplan's syndrome?
5 List the five different conditions associated with exposure to asbestos.

Answers

4 Definition of the terms sarcoidosis, pneumoconiosis, the occupations associated with the commoner pneumoconioses, and a description of Caplan's syndrome

i *Sarcoidosis* is defined as a systemic disease of unknown aetiology associated with an unusual immune reaction and an inflammatory infiltrate of T_4 helper lymphocytes and macrophages and the formation of non-caseating granulomata in many tissues. It tends to resolve spontaneously or heal by fibrosis.

Many organs may be affected by sarcoidosis. From a respiratory point of view the condition tends to affect the thoracic lymph nodes and interstitium of the lungs.

ii *The pneumoconioses* are defined as a group of ILD resulting from chronic exposure to inorganic dust. The most common pneumoconioses are coalworker's pneumoconiosis, silicosis and asbestosis.

iii   *Occupation and the pneumoconioses:*

● Coal worker's   Coal mining
pneumoconiosis

● Silicosis   Tunnelling, quarrying, foundry and
                                   pottery work

● Asbestosis   Asbestos mining and processing,
                                   building industry, shipyard and
                                   ship's engine room work

iv   *Caplan's syndrome* is the association in coal miners of large
round lung opacities with rheumatoid arthritis, a high titre of
rheumatoid factor, and often subcutaneous nodules. Occasionally
the nodules in the lung cavitate or coalesce to form dense fibrosis.

5   The five different conditions associated with exposure to asbestos

● *Mesothelioma.* A slow growing fibrous malignant tumour of
the pleura or peritoneum occurring only in persons who have
been exposed to asbestos.
● *Pleural plaques.* Areas of pleural calcification that are usually
an incidental finding on a chest x-ray.
● *Pleural effusion.*
● *Asbestosis.* A form of ILD associated with a neutrophil-
macrophage alveolitis (see page 267).
● *Carcinoma of the bronchus.* In non-smokers, exposure to
asbestos is associated with an increased incidence of
adenocarcinoma. In smokers the commonest tumours are those
associated with smoking, namely squamous cell and small cell,
both of which occur about six times more frequently than in
smokers not exposed to asbestos.

Diagnosis (i)
Questions

The specific diagnosis in a case of ILD depends upon the following
factors: the history, the physical findings, the distribution of any
abnormal shadowing on a chest x-ray, the results of other specific
investigations, and the histology obtained by bronchoalveolar lavage
and lung biopsy.
With the aim of providing a clinically logical framework for
discussion, these diagnostic parameters have been used to
construct the following questions and answers.
6i   *The history.* Bearing in mind the spectrum of diseases
covered by the term ILD, put on your 'ILD or pulmonary fibrosis
hat' and list the specific direct questions that should be asked to
elucidate the diagnosis in a case of suspected ILD.
   ii   What are the typical symptoms of ILD?
7   *The physical findings.* Describe the main signs of ILD.

Answers

6i   Your 'ILD or pulmonary fibrosis hat' and the specific questions that should be asked in a case of suspected ILD

The point of these questions is to elucidate occupational or recreational exposure to inorganic or organic dusts, and very occasionally drugs. In most cases chronic exposure is necessary for the development of the condition, varying from a few months in the case of extrinsic allergic alveolitis and asbestosis, to many years in the case of coal worker's pneumoconiosis and silicosis.

Always ask specifically about:

● *Occupation and exposure to inorganic dusts* such as coal dust, silica in quarrying, tunnelling, the foundry and pottery industries, or exposure to asbestos in an asbestos mine or processing factory, in the building industry, in a shipyard or as a ship's engine room worker.

● *Occupation and hobbies leading to exposure to organic dusts*, for instance farm work leading to exposure to hay, bird fancying, or occasionally even exposure to the fungal dusts associated with such occupations as growing mushrooms in confined spaces (mushroom worker's lung).

● *Drugs*. If suspected, a full history of past and present medications should be sought.

Comment

The importance of obtaining a history of exposure to dust is amply illustrated by the following case history. Mr J-P, a 44 year old stockbroker, attended the clinic with a 3 month history of breathlessness on exertion, particularly at weekends. Examination and spirometry were normal but chest x-ray showed slight bilateral reticular infiltration of the middle and upper lung fields. He denied any exposure to inhaled dusts. However, when seen again 3 weeks later he said that as a result of the direct questioning at his first visit he now realised that his breathlessness developed on Saturday and Sunday afternoons, about 4 hours after helping his wife bag hay for selling to children in her pet shop.

The history and x-ray findings suggest a mild form of farmer's lung. Serum antibodies against *Micropolyspora faeni* were weakly positive. The patient's condition and x-ray changes resolved as soon as he gave up working with hay.

6ii   The typical symptoms of ILD

● *Initially* the symptoms are *fatigue and breathlessness on exertion* due to lack of oxygenation of the blood. Any cough is usually non-productive.

● *Eventually breathlessness occurs at rest*. Because the airways are patent and unobstructed usually the accessory muscles are not used. Late in the disease patients may develop oedema of the legs due to cor pulmonale.

7   The main signs of ILD

● The most common sign is *tachypnoea*.
● *Clubbing* of the fingers and/or *late inspiratory crackles* tend to occur with cryptogenic fibrosing alveolitis, fibrosing alveolitis associated with the collagenoses, extrinsic allergic alveolitis and asbestosis, but not with sarcoidosis.
● *Cyanosis* occurs as the disease develops.

Diagnosis (ii)
Questions

8   *The chest x-ray*. Describe the typical distribution on a chest x-ray of the abnormal shadowing found with the commoner types of ILD. For example what is the typical distribution of coal worker's pneumoconiosis, silicosis, asbestosis, sarcoidosis, extrinsic allergic alveolitis and cryptogenic fibrosing alveolitis? In addition what is the typical chest x-ray distribution of the non-interstitial lung diseases, bronchiectasis, post-primary pulmonary tuberculosis and lymphangitis carcinomatosis?

9   *Other specific investigations*. Briefly describe the pattern of results you might expect from the following investigations.
i   Spirometry.
ii   Diffusing capacity.
iii   Blood gases.
iv   Radioactive gallium scanning.
v   Serum angiotensin converting enzyme (SACE).
In the cases of diffusing capacity, radioactive gallium scanning and SACE also describe the underlying principles and factors upon which the investigation is based.

Answers

8   The typical distribution on a chest x-ray of the commoner types of ILD, bronchiectasis, post-primary pulmonary tuberculosis and lymphangitis carcinomatosis

Diagnosis is aided by appreciating that typically many of these conditions are associated with a characteristic distribution of abnormal reticular or nodular shadowing in the lung fields of a chest x-ray.

Middle and upper lobes

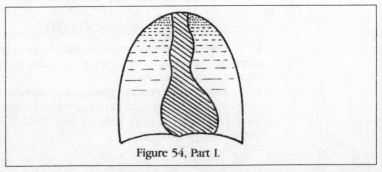

Figure 54, Part I.

- Sarcoidosis
- Extrinsic allergic alveolitis
- Coal worker's pneumoconiosis
- Silicosis
- Post-primary tuberculosis

Lower lobes

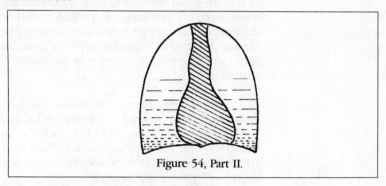

Figure 54, Part II.

- Cryptogenic fibrosing alveolitis
- Fibrosing alveolitis associated with the collagenoses
- Bronchiectasis
- Asbestosis
- Lymphangitis carcinomatosis

NOTE: Lymphangitis carcinomatosis is malignant infiltration of the lymphatics within the lung. As the lymphatics drain to the hila it sometimes appears as a flare radiating out from the hila.

9 Other specific investigations

i *Spirometry.* As the condition develops spirometry typically shows a restrictive pattern with reduction of vital capacity but maintenance of FEV_1 as a percentage of the vital capacity.

ii *Diffusing capacity.* The diffusion of gas into the lungs depends upon firstly factors that are or can be made constant, and secondly factors that vary with the condition of the patient and can be exploited to yield information about disease of the lung. These two types of factors may be summarised as follows:

Constant factors

- The solubility and diffusibility of the gas.
- The difference between the pressure of the gas in the alveoli and in the blood.

Factors that vary with the patient and the disease of the lung

- The area, thickness and quality of the alveolar membrane.
- The volume of blood in the lungs into which the gas has to diffuse.

● Matching of ventilation to perfusion (the importance of this is discussed on page 261).
● The haemoglobin value. Allowance for this has to be made because the avidity of the gas for haemoglobin will be affected by any anaemia or polycythaemia.

In practice the gas used for diffusion studies is carbon monoxide. In ILD the main cause of impaired CO-diffusing capacity is mismatching of ventilation to perfusion, and only to a lesser extent thickening and damage of the alveolar membrane. Nonetheless measurement of CO-diffusing capacity gives useful information about the severity and progress of the disease and any response to treatment.

iii   *Blood gases*. Because of reduced diffusing capacity, typically these show mild hypoxia and a low $PaCO_2$ as the patient tends to hyperventilate and blow off CO_2 from the sense of dyspnoea induced by the changed mechanics of the lung (see page 261). rather than because of hypoxaemia. As the disease progresses, the degree of hypoxaemia increases.

iv   *Radioactive gallium scanning with gallium-67*. Gallium is avidly taken up by the activated macrophages found in the lung in many types of ILD. The test cannot therefore be used to differentiate between the various types of ILD, but is useful for monitoring the activity of a disease within a single patient. However, its use is limited by the fact that the isotope costs more than £100 per dose.

v   *Serum angiotensin converting enzyme (SACE)*. This enzyme is normally found in the endothelial cells of the pulmonary capillaries. In addition *it is elaborated by the cells of the sarcoid granuloma*. SACE is elevated in about 60% of cases of active sarcoidosis, but has a false positive rate of about 10%. It is therefore not a good diagnostic test, but may be used to monitor disease activity in established cases of sarcoidosis.

Diagnosis (iii): the histology
Question

10i   What is bronchoalveolar lavage?
ii   What are the approximate numbers and predominant types of inflammatory cells found round the alveolus of normal individuals?
iii   Which inflammatory cells are thought to cause the tissue damage associated with ILD?
iv   What are the predominant types of inflammatory cells found in sarcoidosis and extrinsic allergic alveolitis on the one hand and cryptogenic fibrosing alveolitis and asbestosis on the other?
v   Draw a diagram showing the main histological features of (a) the normal alveolar wall and interstitium, and (b) the typical changes that occur in these structures with ILD.

Answer

10   The histology of ILD

i   *Bronchoalveolar lavage (BAL)* is a technique in which a bronchoscope is wedged into a distal bronchus and aliquots of warm sterile saline are used to recover inflammatory cells from the distal respiratory tract. The recovered cells are representative of the inflammatory process within the alveoli.

ii   *The inflammatory cells in a normal alveolus.* In normal individuals there are approximately 80 inflammatory cells per alveolus. Ninety per cent of these are macrophages derived from blood monocytes. The remainder are T lymphocytes with a small number of B lymphocytes. Except in smokers, neutrophils are rare.

iii   *Tissue damaging cells within the alveolus in ILD.* Because they release toxic oxidising agents such as OH• groups, and tissue damaging proteolytic enzymes such as elastase, *neutrophils followed by macrophages* are the most damaging cells in the vicinity of the alveolus.
    In addition macrophages release substances that attract fibroblasts leading to the deposition of collagen.

iv   *The predominant type of inflammatory cells found in ILD* varies with the condition. For example:

Disease	Type of alveolitis
● Sarcoidosis and extrinsic allergic alveolitis	Lymphocyte, macrophage and non-caseating granulomata. In sarcoidosis the lymphocytes are T4 helper, and in extrinsic allergic alveolitis T8 suppressor
● Cryptogenic fibrosing alveolitis and asbestosis	Neutrophil and macrophage

v   *Diagram showing the typical histological changes associated with ILD.* As illustrated on the next page, the inflammatory process is associated with enlargement and desquamation of the flat type I alveolar cells through which gases diffuse and their replacement by thicker surfactant producing type II cells and bronchiolar cells that have migrated down from the airways. Within the interstitium the inflammatory process leads to an accumulation of fibroblasts and the production of collagen.

Pulmonary sarcoidosis

Questions

11   How is pulmonary sarcoidosis staged on chest x-ray? What in general terms is the relationship of the x-ray changes to the symptoms and prognosis of the condition?

12   What are the indications for treating pulmonary sarcoidosis? How is it treated and how is the response to treatment monitored?

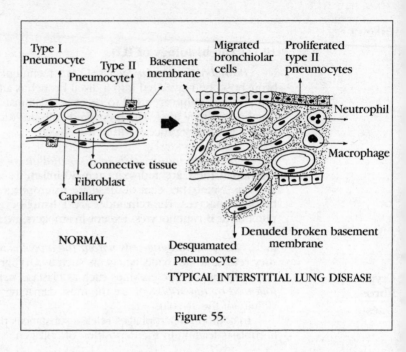

Figure 55.

Answers

11   Chest x-ray changes

Sarcoidosis has been defined and the pathological changes
associated with it have been discussed in the answers to the
preceding questions. By convention the chest x-ray changes
associated with the condition are divided into three stages.
Although this is an aid to learning and thinking it does not
necessarily imply temporal progression, some patients for instance,
presenting with stage III disease that resolves spontaneously.

Stage I: bilateral hilar lymphadenopathy with clear lung fields,
although at a histological level granulomata may be found in the
interstitium of the lung. About 60% of patients fall into this
category.
Stage II: bilateral hilar lymphadenopathy together with reticular
infiltration of the lung fields, particularly in the middle and upper
zones. About 25% of patients are in this category.
Stage III: diffuse reticular infiltration of the lung fields without hilar
lymphadenopathy.

Relationship of staging to symptoms and prognosis

It is important to appreciate that in general the density of the
infiltration seen on chest x-ray correlates poorly with symptoms
and outcome. Nonetheless stage I disease is rarely associated with
respiratory symptoms and has an 80% likelihood of resolving
spontaneously within 2 years. Stage II disease also has a 70–80%

likelihood of spontaneous resolution, and in many cases is associated with surprisingly few symptoms. Exercise limiting breathlessness, a chronic course, and a guarded prognosis are more likely in the category of stage III disease associated with dense irregular mottling in the lung fields and linear shadows extending from the hila.

12   Treatment

Because it has an 80% likelihood of spontaneous resolution, specific treatment is not usually required for stage I sarcoidosis of the lung. Breathlessness on exertion is the main indication for treatment of the other stages. Prednisolone 30 mg daily is given for 4-6 weeks, thereafter reducing to the lowest necessary maintenance dose for as long as the disease is active. Treatment is monitored both subjectively by the response of the patient's symptoms, and objectively by measuring diffusing capacity.

Cryptogenic fibrosing alveolitis (CFA) (also known as idiopathic pulmonary fibrosis—IPF)

Questions

13   By way of introduction, in a few sentences summarise the clinical and radiological features of CFA. What types of inflammatory cells are involved in this type of alveolitis?

14   CFA is thought to have an immunological basis. Very briefly, in a sentence or two, describe what the basis of this immunological mechanism is thought to be.

15   At a histological level, the changes within the alveolus in CFA are described as spanning a spectrum. Very briefly, in a sentence or two describe the histology of the two ends of this spectrum. Why is it important from a clinical point of view to appreciate the spectrum of changes?

16i   What is usually the clinical clue differentiating CFA from bronchiectasis?

   ii   What are the three main late complications of CFA?

17   How is CFA treated? In percentage terms what is the likelihood of response?

18   What are the special or distinguishing features of the fibrosing alveolitis associated with the collagenoses?

Answers

13   Clinical and radiological features of CFA

In general terms the criteria for diagnosing CFA have been covered in the answers to previous questions and may be summarised as a *negative history of exposure to inhaled dusts, and either the whole (in up to 70% of cases) or part of a clinical triad* consisting of breathlessness and cough without sputum, clubbing of the fingers, and bilateral late inspiratory crackles. Usually these features are associated with an abnormal infiltrate in the lower lung fields on chest x-ray, although occasionally the x-ray may appear normal. Histology obtained from bronchoalveolar lavage and lung biopsy shows a neutrophil-macrophage alveolitis.

14   The immunological basis of CFA

The aetiology of CFA is not known, but may be autoimmune involving immune complexes of antigen/antibody that activate alveolar macrophages.

15   The histological spectrum of changes within the alveolus in CFA

This is from a fibrotic or 'mural' more chronic type at one end of the spectrum to a 'desquamative' more acute cellular type at the other end. The clinical importance of the two types is that being 'active' the desquamative type tends to respond to corticosteroid therapy whereas the 'inactive' fibrotic types do not.

16   Clinical differentiation between CFA and bronchiectasis; late complications of CFA

i   With the exception of sputum production, CFA and bronchiectasis often present with similar clinical and chest x-ray findings. However, in CFA any cough is typically non-productive, whereas in most but not every case of bronchiectasis, sputum production is usually copious, often measurable in terms of a quarter or half or more of a cup per day.

ii   The three main late complications of CFA are
• Death from type I respiratory failure (hypoxaemia)
• Cor pulmonale
• Up to 10% likelihood of developing carcinoma of the bronchus

17   The treatment of CFA

This is with oral corticosteroids. Usually *a trial* of prednisolone 60 mg daily is given for a month, reducing to the lowest necessary maintenance dose in those who respond, generally 10–15 mg daily. In those who do not respond the drug should be withdrawn. Cyclophosphamide occasionally helps these cases.

The likelihood of objective response is 15–20%, with subjective improvement in a further 30%.

18   Fibrosing alveolitis associated with collagenoses such as rheumatoid arthritis, systemic lupus erythematosus, scleroderma, dermatomyositis and polyarteritis nodosa

This presents a similar clinical and histological picture to CFA although there is usually clinical evidence of the underlying systemic disease. The course of the lung disease tends to be more slowly progressive, and response to corticosteroids less than with CFA.

Extrinsic allergic alveolitis (EAA) (also known as hypersensitivity pneumonitis)
Questions

19   By way of introduction, in a few sentences summarise the clinical and radiological features of EAA. What types of cells are involved in this type of alveolitis?

20   What types of hypersensitivity reaction are thought to be involved in EAA?

21   What blood test should be asked for to support a diagnosis of, for example, farmer's lung or bird fancier's lung?

22   How is EAA treated?

Answers

19   Clinical and radiological features of EAA

A list of the commoner forms of EAA and the principles underlying their diagnosis have been covered in the answers to the previous questions, and may be summarised as (a) a positive history of exposure to an inhaled organic dust, (b) breathlessness and the clinical picture described below, (c) an infiltrate typically in the middle and upper lung fields of a chest x-ray, and (d) a lymphocyte-macrophage, granulomatous type of alveolitis.

Clinically the picture produced by EAA depends upon the balance between the severity, duration and frequency of exposure to the inhaled organic dust, and host factors within the patient. As a consequence the disease spans a spectrum from intermittent breathlessness of the type illustrated by the case history on page 263 occurring about 4-6 hours after exposure to the dust, to an acute illness with pyrexia, myalgia, more severe breathlessness and late inspiratory crackles, also occurring about 4-6 hours after exposure, to a chronic form of the condition characterised by persistent hypoxaemia, finger clubbing and late inspiratory crackles.

20   The types of hypersensitivity reaction thought to be involved in EAA

It is commonly said that in EAA the main reaction is a type III hypersensitivity reaction of the Arthus type with tissue damaging antigen/IgG antibody immune complexes and the consumption of complement. In support of this is the fact that as with most type III reactions, symptoms usually begin 4-6 hours after exposure to the antigen. However, immune complexes have not been demonstrated in the lungs, and the occurrence of granulomata suggests that type IV cell mediated hypersensitivity is also involved.

21   The blood test that should be asked for in a case of suspected EAA

Specific IgG antibodies to the inhaled dust are usually measured, but the diagnosis rests more on a history of exposure and response to avoidance of the dust than on the demonstration of a positive titre. Thus absence of the antibody does not exclude the diagnosis, whilst its presence implies only previous exposure, positive titres being found in many asymptomatic previously exposed individuals.

22   The treatment of EAA

This takes two forms:
- *Avoidance of the antigen* by getting rid of any birds or by changing occupation.
- *Corticosteroids*. Patients with severe symptoms should be given a trial of prednisolone 40 mg daily, reducing, and if possible stopping the drug after 4-6 weeks. In chronic severe cases the changes within the lung may be irreversible and unresponsive to treatment.

Further Reading

Crystal RG, Bitterman PB, Rennard SI, Hance AJ, Keogh BA (1984). Interstitial lung diseases of unknown cause. *N.Engl.J.Med. 310*, 154-66; 235-44.

Case O # Another Case of Breathlessness: Mr P-S, aged 72 years

A happily married retired electrician living in his own small detached bungalow.

History of present condition

For 3 months prior to presentation this elderly man had exprienced breathlessness on exertion such as working in the garden or climbing slopes. In addition, although he felt reasonably well he volunteered that during the previous year he had experienced three episodes of chest infection with temperature and cough productive of yellow sputum, and that on each occasion he had received a course of an antibiotic.

Apart from breathlessness on exertion, more recently he had noticed that his voice had become rather hoarse, and that during the last 2 weeks he had coughed a little blood on four or five occasions.

Past medical history

No previous illness or operations.

Relevant direct questions

Appetite: poor with associated 14 lb weight loss in the previous month.
Sputum: minimal white mucoid sputum flecked with blood in the previous 2 weeks.
Smoking: two small cigars per day for 10 years. Prior to that 20 cigarettes per day for approximately 40 years.

Examination

Big well looking elderly man in whom clinical examination was normal except for slight hoarseness, clubbing of the fingers and reduced breath sounds over the front and back of the left upper chest. BP 150/95 lying and standing. Spirometry, $FEV_1/VC = 1.2/2.2$ (55%).

Mr P-S, haemoptysis, finger clubbing and associated conditions

Questions

1   What two diagnoses are suggested by the history and physical findings?

2   What commonly ordered investigation would you have asked for immediately to confirm your suspicions? What do you think it might have shown in Mr P-S's case?
3   Mr P-S complained of coughing blood. List the main causes of haemoptysis, classifying them according to underlying mechanism.
4   Mr P-S had finger clubbing. List the main causes of finger clubbing, classifying them according to underlying mechanism.
5   The following conditions are among the causes of haemoptysis or finger clubbing. Write two or three lines about each, describing their essentials:
i   Goodpasture's syndrome
ii   Wegener's granulomatosis
iii Tetralogy of Fallot
iv   Eisenmenger's syndrome

Answers

1   The diagnosis suggested by the history and physical findings in Mr P-S's case

The combination of recurrent chest infections, breathlessness, hoarseness of the voice, haemoptysis, anorexia, weight loss, a past history of heavy cigarette smoking, clubbing of the fingers, and signs in the upper part of the left lung all suggest that Mr P-S was suffering from carcinoma of the bronchus, probably with involvement of the left recurrent laryngeal nerve as it passes under the aortic arch.

However, but for the hoarse voice, it was also possible that he was suffering from pulmonary tuberculosis.

The results of the spirometry, $FEV_1/VC = 1.2/2.2$, 55%, indicate that in addition Mr S-A was also suffering from chronic obstructive airways disease. The interpretation of the results of spirometry is discussed on pages 222–223.

2   The investigation that should have been asked for immediately to confirm the diagnosis

This was a chest x-ray which is abnormal in 95% of cases of carcinoma of the bronchus. The changes that are likely to be seen are listed in the answer to question 13 on page 285.

In Mr P-S's case chest x-ray showed a large carcinoma 4½ cm in diameter in the left upper lobe together with enlargement of the left hilum.

Further history

Ten days after his initial presentation Mr P-S developed a swelling at the medial end of the right clavicle. Needle aspiration of this revealed carcinoma cells. He was treated with a course of palliative radiotherapy to the clavicle and to the lung. Three months later an area of induration developed in the cutaneous tissues over the abdomen. Needle aspiration of this yielded malignant cells. Within a few days the liver became enlarged, hard and craggy, and 3 weeks later he died.

3   The main causes of haemoptysis

Pulmonary

- Carcinoma of the bronchus
- Pulmonary embolus
- Tuberculosis
- Bronchiectasis
- Goodpasture's syndrome
- Wegener's granulomatosis
- Bronchial adenoma (80% carcinoid)

Pulmonary congestion

- Left ventricular failure
- In association with mitral stenosis

Bleeding disorders

- Blood dyscrasias
- Anticoagulant therapy

An isolated episode

- Possibly associated with a chest infection or cough, in an otherwise healthy person.

NOTE:

- *Pneumonia.* Klebsiella and legionella pneumonia may be associated with haemoptysis. In other forms of pneumonia frank haemoptysis should arouse suspicion of an underlying lesion such as bronchiectasis or a carcinoma.
- *Chronic bronchitis and emphysema.* Although haemoptysis may occur occasionally in these conditions its occurrence should arouse suspicion of an underlying lesion such as carcinoma.

4   The main causes of finger clubbing

Pulmonary

- Carcinoma of the bronchus
- Cryptogenic fibrosing alveolitis
- Extrinsic allergic alveolitis
- Asbestosis
- Suppuration:
  Tuberculosis
  Bronchiectasis
  Lung abscess
  Empyema
- Fibrocystic disease

Cardiovascular

- Infective endocarditis
- Cyanotic heart disease with right to left shunt, e.g.
  Fallot's tetralogy
  Eisenmenger's syndrome

Liver and bowel disease (occasionally)

- Cirrhosis
- Ulcerative colitis
- Crohn's disease

NOTE: Finger clubbing is not a feature of chronic bronchitis and emphysema.

5   Conditions causing haemoptysis or finger clubbing

i   *Goodpasture's syndrome* is a triad of unknown aetiology characterised by pulmonary haemorrhage, glomerulonephritis and antibodies to lung and glomerular basement membrane. Typically the patients are young men. It is associated with recurrent haemoptysis and renal failure that in many cases requires regular dialysis or renal transplantation.

ii   *Wegener's granulomatosis* is a condition of unknown aetiology characterised by necrotising vasculitis and granulomatous inflammation affecting the lungs, sinuses, kidneys and often other organs. It is associated with haemoptysis, pneumonitis and renal failure that is often potentially fatal. The eyes and nervous system may also be involved.

iii   *Fallot's tetralogy.* See page 198.

iv   *Eisenmenger's syndrome.* See page 197.

Chapter 19
Carcinoma of the Bronchus

Aetiology; cell types

Questions

1   Considering all the organs in the body, which is the commonest carcinoma in men and in women respectively? Approximately how many people die of carcinoma of the bronchus each year?

2   List and write notes on the main aetiological factors concerned with the development of carcinoma of the bronchus. Which of the main components of tobacco smoke is thought to be carcinogenic?

3   List the various histological types of carcinoma of the bronchus, and write a few words of description about the main characteristics of the cells of each type. In percentage terms what is the approximate proportion of each? What is the approximate cell doubling time of each?

Answers

1   The commonest carcinoma in men and in women, and the number of people that die each year of carcinoma of the bronchus

Carcinoma of the bronchus is the commonest carcinoma in men. In women carcinoma of the breast is commonest, although carcinoma of the bronchus is rapidly becoming as common as a result of increased smoking among women.

Each year about 35 000 people die of carcinoma of the bronchus in Britain, and in the United States about 120 000.

2   The main aetiological factors in carcinoma of the bronchus and the carcinogenic component of tobacco smoke

●   *Smoking* is suggested by the direct relationship between the number of cigarettes smoked per day or the number smoked in a person's lifetime and the likelihood of dying of carcinoma of the bronchus, and also by the decrease of this likelihood when smoking is stopped, although the risk never returns to the level found among people who have never smoked.

Pipe and cigar smoking is less carcinogenic than cigarettes.

It is thought that tar is the carcinogenic component of tobacco smoke.

● *Occupation*. The risk of carcinoma of the bronchus is increased by exposure to:

a   Asbestos—increased risk × 6.

b   Radon in pitchblende and uranium mines.

c   Polycyclic aromatic hydrocarbons in gas and coke oven works.

d   Nickel, chromium, arsenic.

● *Air pollution*. Although carcinoma of the bronchus is more common in urban areas, studies of this point have been confounded by the overwhelming effect of smoking.

● *Scars in the lungs* due to previous tuberculosis or metallic foreign bodies occasionally give rise to adenocarcinoma of the bronchus.

3   The histological types of carcinoma of the bronchus

The WHO classification recognises four main types:

● *Squamous cell (epidermoid)*. About 40-50% of all bronchial carcinoma. Histologically in its well differentiated form it consists of flattened cells that form intercellular bridges and keratin. It tends to spread locally, blocking bronchi, and compared to small cell carcinoma is less likely to metastasise and therefore has a better prognosis. Its cell doubling time is about 90 days.

● *Small cell (oat cell) anaplastic*. About 20% of all bronchial carcinoma. Histologically it consists typically of small cells with scanty cytoplasm and hyperchromatic nuclei. It is highly malignant and metastasises early by blood and lymphatic spread, so that by the time it presents there are micrometastases in over 90% of cases. Its cell doubling time is about 30 days, that is about three times as fast as squamous cell carcinoma.

● *Adenocarcinoma*. About 20-30% of all bronchial carcinoma. It is unrelated to smoking. Histologically it consists of cuboid and columnar cells that contain mucin in about 80% of cases. It is classified into two main types:

a   The regular type derived from bronchial lining.

b   The bronchioloalveolar type thought to be derived from alveolar cells. The bronchioloalveolar type tends to spread transbronchially producing a widespread lesion.

Adenocarcinoma grows very slowly, tends to occur peripheral[and presents with pleural effusion in about 10% of cases. Its cell doubling time is about 190 days.

● *Large cell anaplastic*. About 10% of all bronchial carcinoma. Histologically it consists of cells of different shapes with large nuclei and abundant cytoplasm often containing mucin. It invades locally but metastasises early, so that there are distant metastases i[about half the cases by the time of presentation. Its cell doubling time is about 90 days.

Pathological associations
Questions

4i   In which part of the lungs do the great majority of carcinomas of the bronchus occur, peripherally or proximally?
ii   Which histological types tend to be associated with:
A   Smoking
B   Peripheral location and central location.
C   Early metastases.
D   Cavitation.
E   Hypercalcaemia.
F   Ectopic production of anti-diuretic hormone (ADH) and ACTH.
5   To which five organs does carcinoma of the bronchus show a predilection to metastasise?
6   List the organs outside the chest from which carcinomas tend to produce multiple metastases or 'cannon balls' in the lungs.

Answers

4   Location, and associations with the different cell types of bronchial carcinoma

i   In about 75% of cases bronchial carcinoma occurs centrally, arising from first, second or third order bronchi.

ii
A   Squamous and small cell carcinomas are the types most clearly related to smoking.
B   Adenocarcinoma and large cell anaplastic carcinoma tend to occur peripherally; squamous and small cell carcinomas, the smoking related tumours, tend to occur centrally.
C   The anaplastic carcinomas of the small cell and large cell types tend to metastasise early, but at autopsy, metastases are found in about 50% of all types.
D   Cavities occur most frequently with squamous cell and large cell carcinomas.
E   Hypercalcaemia due to production of a parathormone-like peptide occurs occasionally with squamous cell carcinoma. However, more frequently hypercalcaemia is a result of bone destruction due to bony metastases.
F   Ectopic production of ADH-like and ACTH-like peptides occurs mainly with small cell carcinomas, although occasionally any of peptides produced by bronchial carcinomas may be produced by any of the cell types.

5   The five organs to which carcinoma of the bronchus shows a predilection to spread

- Liver
- Bone
- Lymph nodes of the upper half of the body

- Brain
- Adrenal gland in about 4–8% of cases

6   The organs outside the chest from which carcinomas tend to produce multiple metastases or 'cannon balls' in the lungs

- Kidney (hypernephroma)
- Breast
- Testis, ovary, choriocarcinoma
- Thyroid (follicular)
- Stomach and large bowel

Symptoms and signs
Questions

7   List the various presentations and symptoms of carcinoma of the bronchus.
8   List the signs that may be found in patients with carcinoma of the bronchus.

Answers

7   Presentation and symptoms

Carcinoma of the bronchus may present in many ways, the more common of which include:
- *No symptoms.* In about 5% of cases carcinoma of the bronchus is an incidental finding on a chest x-ray performed for routine or other reasons.
- *Cough.* A *new* persistent cough or *change* in the character of an established cough should always arouse suspicion of carcinoma of the bronchus, especially in smokers.
- *Coughing blood (haemoptysis)* is the only symptom in about 5% of cases.
- *Breathlessness* due to tumour occupying lung tissue, or collapse of a lung or part of a lung, pleural effusion, or lymphangitis carcinomatosis in which tumour spreads via lymphatics in the lung.
- *Weight loss* due to anorexia, diversion of energy to the tumour, and the toxic effects of the tumour upon other tissues.
- *Hoarseness* due to involvement of the left recurrent laryngeal nerve as it passes by the left main bronchus under the aortic arch.
- *Dysphagia.* An occasional symptom due to compression or invasion of the oesophagus.
- *Recurrent or unresolving pneumonia* as a result of a lesion obstructing the drainage of secretions from a bronchus.;
- *Enlargement of lymph nodes* in the upper half of the body, that is of the neck or axilla.
- *Pains in the ribs, spine, pelvis or proximal long bones* due to bony metastases. For reasons that are unknown, metastases are rare in the bones of the more distal parts of the limbs.
- *Pains in the upper abdomen* due to stretching or invasion by

hepatic metastases of the richly innervated capsule of the liver.
● *Pains in the upper chest, shoulder and arm* due to tumour in the superior pulmonary sulcus (*Pancoast tumour*) invading the first and second ribs, and the brachial plexus. Often a tumour in this location is associated with Horner's syndrome.
● *Pains over the wrists and ankles, and less commonly the knees and elbows* due to hypertrophic pulmonary osteoarthropathy, an uncommon distant toxic reaction to a tumour that is usually a peripheral squamous or adenocarcinoma. The condition is associated with clubbing of the fingers, and a toxic periostitis that causes the overlying affected area to be hot, swollen and tender, and can be seen on x-ray as a raised periosteum. Usually it resolves with complete resection of the tumour.
● *Swelling of the face, neck and arms* due to the *superior vena cava syndrome*, caused by tumour obstructing the superior vena cava.
● *Unwellness due to the secretion of peptides* like ADH, ACTH and parathormone.

8   Signs

● *No signs.* A frequent occurrence in patients who present with symptoms such as cough or haemoptysis, or in whom carcinoma is an incidental x-ray finding.
● *Stridor.* A localised wheeze due to narrowing of a large bronchus.
● *Evidence of weight loss* such as loose skin, or clothes that have become too big.
● *Clubbing of the fingers* in about 10% of cases.
● *Signs in the chest* of pleural effusion, collapse or consolidation.
● *Lymphadenopathy* in the upper half of the body.
● *Tenderness to pressure over bony metastases,* or metastases in the liver, which is usually enlarged and craggy to palpation in the presence of advanced metastatic invasion.
● *Swelling of the face, neck and arms* with distension of the veins of the neck due to the superior vena cava syndrome.
● *Hot, tender, swollen wrists and ankles* due to hypertrophic pulmonary osteoarthropathy.
● *Pleural or pericardial rubs* due to invasion of the respective serous membranes.
● *Nodules in the skin* due to cutaneous metastases in about 1% of cases.
● *Atrial fibrillation or atrial flutter* due to invasion of the pericardium.
● *Horner's syndrome.*

Clinical syndromes associated with carcinoma of the bronchus
Questions

9   List the four features of Horner's syndrome. To what is it due in cases of carcinoma of the bronchus?

10   List the neuromyopathies that may occur occasionally with carcinoma of the bronchus. Describe the features that differentiate myasthenia gravis from the myasthenic syndrome of Eaton-Lambert.

11i   Describe ancanthosis nigrans. What are its main causes?

ii   Briefly describe the clinical features of dermatomyositis. Who is likely to develop it? Briefly describe the main biochemical and histological findings of a typical case.

Answers

9   The four features of Horner's syndrome, and its cause in carcinoma of the bronchus

The four features of a fully developed case of Horner's syndrome are:

●   Constriction of the pupil (miosis).
●   Narrowing of the palpable fissure (ptosis).
●   Lack of thermal sweating on the affected side (anhydrosis).
●   A sunken eyeball (enophthalmus).

Horner's syndrome is due to paresis of the sympathetic nerves from the eighth cervical and first and second thoracic ganglia. In carcinoma of the bronchus this results from invasion by tumour, usually a Pancoast tumour in the superior pulmonary sulcus.

10   The neuromyopathies that occur occasionally with carcinoma of the bronchus

These are uncommon distant toxic reactions to carcinoma of the bronchus that occur in about 1% of cases. They include:

●   *Peripheral neuropathy*, which is usually sensory and may be painful, although a mixed sensory/motor neuropathy may also be encountered.
●   *The myasthenic syndrome of Eaton–Lambert*, described below.
●   *Polymyositis or dermatomyositis*, described below.
●   *Subacute cerebellar degeneration* resulting in ataxia.

The distinction between myasthenia gravis and the myasthenic syndrome of Eaton–Lambert

Myasthenia gravis is an autoimmune condition that tends to affect the muscles of the eyes although the muscles of the limbs are also often involved. It is associated with weakness that becomes more marked with sustained or repeated use of the affected muscles, and with antibodies in the serum against the acetylcholine receptors of the motor end plates of striated muscle. It responds to anticholinesterases.

By contrast, with the Eaton-Lambert syndrome the muscles of the eyes are usually spared, and although the patient may complain of weakness, muscle power usually improves with exercise and there are no demonstrable antibodies against acetylcholine receptors. Instead the condition is thought to be due to defective release of acetylcholine as the result of an antibody acting against the calcium channels of the presynaptic nerve ending of the neuromuscular junction. Usually there is no response to anticholinesterases, although there may be a response to guanidine.

11   Acanthosis nigrans and dermatomyositis

i   *Acanthosis nigrans* is a velvety hyperpigmented brown or black elevation of the epidermis that tends to occur in flexures such as the axilla or groin, and also at the umbilicus and nipple area. It may occur congenitally in children, or be stimulated to occur by obesity or abnormal hormonal states such as Cushing's disease. In adults it is often a marker of internal malignancy such as carcinoma of the stomach (60% of such cases), liver, breast, ovary, gut and bronchus.

ii   *Dermatomyositis* is an autoimmune condition that typically presents with an erythematous rash on the face where it may have a butterfly distribution, although often it also involves the V of the neck, the upper trunk and the backs of the fingers and hands. In some cases the upper eyelids take on a purple colour known as a violaceous hue after the purple colour of violets. The proximal mucles of the arms and legs are painful, weak, tender, and usually wasted. Dysphagia may result from involvement of the oesophagus.

The idiopathic form of the condition affects females to males in a 2:1 ratio. In males over 40 there is a 60–70% likelihood of the condition being associated with a carcinoma, particularly of the bronchus or stomach, although in females the site of the tumour may be the breast or ovary. Sometimes, but not always, the condition remits if the tumour is resected.

The main biochemical finding is elevation of the serum enzymes, such as aspartate transaminase and total creatine kinase as a result of release from damaged muscle fibres. Histologically the affected muscles show necrosis of muscle cells, vacuolation and fragmentation of the sarcoplasm, and infiltrates of inflammatory cells such as neutrophils, lymphocytes and plasma cells.

Investigation

Questions

12   List the specific investigations that are often performed in cases of carcinoma of the bronchus.

Include a note about the anaemias that may be found, including a brief description of leuco-erythroblastic anaemia.

In what percentage of cases of carcinoma of the bronchus do the following investigations yield positive results: chest x-ray, sputum cytology, bronchoscopy?

Why is bronchoscopy performed? What are the bronchoscopic criteria used to decide whether or not a lesion is operable?

What are the currently accepted indications for CT scanning and mediastinoscopy?

What simple clinical tests are used to decide whether or not a patient will tolerate pneumonectomy without being permanently breathless?

13   Describe the commoner changes seen on chest x-ray in cases of carcinoma of the bronchus.

Answers

12   Specific investigations

● *Full blood count.* Occasionally this may reveal an anaemia due to *chronic illness suppressing the bone marrow.* Usually this is a normochromic anaemia, although if there is defective incorporation of iron into the developing red cells it may be microcytic, whilst if there is depression of nuclear development it may be macrocytic.

Rarely a *leuco-erythroblastic anaemia* may occur as a result of direct infiltration of the bone marrow by tumour cells. This is characterised by nucleated therefore abnormally early red blood cells together with abnormally early white blood cells being pushed out into the peripheral blood. It may be caused by carcinomas other than the bronchus, and also by myelofibrosis.

● *Serum electrolytes. Hyponatraemia* may result from inappropriate ADH secretion, or from Addison's disease due to destruction of the adrenal glands.

Hypokalaemia may result from secretion of ACTH.

● *Chest x-ray* is abnormal in 95% of cases of carcinoma of the bronchus. In 5% of cases it may appear normal because the lesion is too small to be seen, or is central and hidden within the mediastinum.

● *Sputum cytology.* In expert hands three samples sent freshly to the laboratory yield positive results in up to 80% of cases. However, because the cells are from superficial degenerative parts of the tumour in up to 10% of cases the cell type reported is different to that found by formal biopsy.

● *Fibreoptic bronchoscopy.* This is performed for two main purposes:

a   To confirm the diagnosis by formal biopsy.

b   To assess operability. The main criteria of this are:
     The proximal 2 cm of the main bronchus should be free of tumour.
     The carina must appear sharp and free from widening due to underlying malignant lymphadenopathy.

With modern methods of tissue sampling that include bronchial brushings and washings, and transbronchial biopsy, fibreoptic bronchoscopy yields a positive diagnosis in up to 80% of cases.

● *Biopsy of any abnormal tissue* such as an abnormally palpable lymph node or suspicious subcutaneous nodule. When a pleural effusion is present, fluid may be withdrawn and sent for cytology and a pleural biopsy performed.

● *Computerised tomography.* If available this is performed:

a   Following bronchoscopy, in all patients with

bronchoscopically apparently operable lesions to ascertain whether there is mediastinal spread that might contraindicate surgery.

b   Whether or not surgery is contemplated, for cases in which it is difficult to make a diagnosis.

● *Mediastinoscopy*. The purpose of this is to assess whether there is metastatic spread to the mediastinum:

a   In apparently otherwise operable cases in which mediastinal spread is suspected, and CT scanning is not available.

b   To determine by biopsy whether or not an abnormality seen in the mediastinum on a CT scan is benign or malignant.

c   Occasionally mediastinoscopy is also performed in cases in which operation is not contemplated because the mediastinum is clearly abnormal on chest x-ray, but a biopsy proven diagnosis is required and bronchoscopy is normal.

● *Isotope liver, brain and bone scans*. Experience has shown that these are helpful only in identifying metastases in the presence of symptoms and signs.

● *Tests to assess fitness for operation*. Surgery is contraindicated if it will leave the patient permanently short of breath. Rough guides to fitness for pneumonectomy are:

a $FEV_1 > 1.2$ litres.

b   Ability to climb two to three flights of stairs without undue breathlessness.

13   The commoner chest x-ray changes in carcinoma of the bronchus

● *A peripheral lesion*

a   Carcinoma is suggested if there are spicules radiating out into the surrounding tissue or if the lesion is hazy. Statistically adenocarcinoma and large cell anaplastic carcinomas are more common peripherally.

b   Occasionally a clearly demarcated nodule or coin lesion is seen; 30% of these are malignant. They should therefore be resected if the patient is fit and not too old.

c   Occasionally carcinoma of the bronchus may arise at more than one site, presenting on x-ray with multiple round shadows or 'cannon balls'.

● *Enlargement of a hilum* due to a central tumour, often with extension out into the surrounding lung tissue. Statistically, these tumours are likely to be squamous cell or small cell anaplastic carcinomas associated with smoking.

● *A mass containing a cavity*. Statistically these are most likely to be squamous cell or large cell anaplastic carcinoma. However, pyogenic abscesses and tuberculous lesions often cavitate.

● *Collapse of all or part of a lung, consolidation, or pleural effusion*.

● *Lymphadenopathy and widening of the upper half of the mediastinum*.

● *A raised diaphragm* due to involvement and paralysis of the phrenic nerve, or to collapse of part of a lung.

- *Bony metastases in the ribs, clavicles or upper end of the humerus.*
- *Lymphangitis carcinomatosis.* A reticular pattern in the lung field that mimics pulmonary fibrosis, or streaky shadows extending out from the hila due to spread of tumour along lymphatics.

Treatment
Questions

14i For which histological types of carcinoma of the bronchus is surgery indicated, and for which is radiotherapy and chemotherapy indicated?
   ii What is the 5 year survival for patients treated with surgery?
15 List the contraindications to surgical treatment of carcinoma of the bronchus. What is the likelihood of an apparently operable lesion being found to be inoperable at thoracotomy?
16 What are the indications for (i) curative radiotherapy and (ii) palliative radiotherapy in cases of carcinoma of the bronchus? How is malignant pleural effusion treated?

Answers

14   Treatment and histological type; 5 year survival after surgery

i   Unless contraindicated for the reasons given in the answer to the next question, *in a fit patient with a bronchoscopically operable lesion surgery is the treatment of choice for squamous cell, adenocarcinoma and large cell carcinoma of the bronchus.*
   Because it has metastasised in more than 90% of cases by the time of diagnosis, *surgery is not indicated in the treatment of small cell anaplastic carcinoma.* However, with this type of tumour the combination of radiotherapy and chemotherapy prolongs life, and cures about 7% of cases.

ii   *Five year survival of patients treated with surgery:*
- The prognosis is best with small peripheral lesions. Surgery of squamous cell carcinoma of this type yields a 5 year survival of about 50%.
- However, overall only about 25% of histologically suitable carcinomas of the bronchus prove to be operable, and of those operated upon only 25% survive 5 years. Thus overall only about 6% (25% of 25%) of those with tumours of a histological type suitable for surgery survive 5 years.

15   Contraindications to surgery

- Small cell anaplastic carcinoma.
- An unfit patient or a patient in whom surgery would result in permanent breathlessness.
- Invasion of adjoining structures.
- Distant metastases.

Unfitness is indicated by:
- Shortness of breath on slight exertion. It has already been mentioned that the ability to climb two to three flights of stairs without undue breathlessness is a rough guide to fitness.
- Poor physical state.
- $FEV_1 < 1.2$ litres for patients requiring pneumonectomy.
- Cardiac failure.
- Age. A relative contraindication, surgery rarely being attempted after age 76-78 years.
- Pancoast tumour. Also a relative contraindication.

Invasion of adjoining structures including evidence of spread to involve:

The phrenic nerve	The vena cava
The oesophagus	The mediastinum
The pericardium	

Pleural effusion

Despite careful selection, at thoracotomy 8-10% of cases are found to be inoperable.
NOTE: Enlargement of the hilum on the same side as a lesion does not necessarily mean that a tumour is inoperable.

16   Radiotherapy.

i   *Curative radiotherapy* (5-6000 rads over 5-6 weeks) may be attempted in cases that appear suitable for surgery but for:
- Refusal by the patient to consent to surgery.
- Small lesions too central to be amenable to surgery.

However, whereas the 5 year survival after surgery for small peripheral highly operable lesions is about 50%, after radiotherapy it is only about 5%.

ii   *Palliative radiotherapy* (approximately 3000 rads). In the absence of curative surgery or radiotherapy, carcinoma of the bronchus is uniformly fatal. Since often it induces lethargy and prolongs life by only a matter of weeks, and since it can be given only once to any particular area and by definition is not curative, palliative radiotherapy is usually reserved for the treatment of unpleasant symptoms such as:
- Breathlessness due to collapse in a lung, or to tumour bulk.
- Haemoptysis.
- Localised skeletal pain, including Pancoast tumour.
- Superior vena cava syndrome.

Malignant pleural effusion. Radiotherapy is ineffective in the treatment of malignant pleural effusion which should be treated by total drainage and injection of a sclerosing agent such as tetracycline or mepacrine, talc or a cytotoxic such as thiotepa or bleomycin.

Further Reading

Crofton J, Douglas A (1981). *Respiratory Diseases*, 3rd edition. Blackwell Scientific Publications, Oxford. Chapter 34, lung cancer.

Weatherall DJ, Ledingham JGG, Warrell DA (eds) (1987). *Oxford Textbook of Medicine*, 2nd edition. Oxford University Press, Oxford. Tumours of the lung, mediastinum and pleura, pp 15.145-58.

Case P

Old Soldiers Never Die:
Colonel B-S, aged 52 years

A retired paratroop officer who currently breeds rare prize ducks.

History of present condition

A previously fit non-smoking retired army officer who on the day of admission suddenly became very unwell with fever and feelings of malaise, aching of the limbs and shivers.

Past medical and family history

Nil of note.

Examination

6ft 5in, strong sandy haired pyrexial middle-aged man with a flushed complexion.
Temperature 38.5°C, pulse 100 regular, respiratory rate 24, BP 140/85 lying and standing.
Examination normal except for dullness to percussion, increased tactile and vocal fremitus, a few late inspiratory crackles and bronchial breathing at the base of the left lung.

Colonel B-S
Questions

1   What do you think the diagnosis was in this case?
2   In view of the colonel's occupation, what specific test, apart from a chest x-ray, would you have ordered to elucidate the underlying or particular cause of his condition?
3   In view of the possible underlying condition, how would you have treated him?

Answers

1   Diagnosis

The history of an acute febrile illness and the physical findings of consolidation at the base of the left lung suggest that Colonel B-S was suffering from pneumonia.

2   Specific test

The history of breeding birds raised the possibility that the pneumonia in this case was due to ornithosis (psittacosis). The colonel was unable to produce any sputum for culture, but paired samples of serum taken 12 days apart showed a sixfold increase of antibodies against *Chlamydia psittaci*, confirming the diagnosis.

3   Treatment

Because psittacosis was suspected from the outset, the colonel was treated with oral tetracycline 500 mg four times daily for a week. He made a good recovery. Psittacosis is discussed later in Chapter 20.

Chapter 20
Pneumonia

Definition; clinical features; investigation

Questions

1 Define the term 'pneumonia'.
2 What organisms cause pneumonia in the community outside hospital in Britain? What are roughly the percentages or proportions of each?
3 Discuss the spectrum of
i The symptoms.
ii The signs that occur with the bacterial pneumonias. What are the classical signs of consolidation of the lung?
iii What are the main complications of pneumonia?
4 How is pneumonia investigated? What results might be expected?

Answers

1 Definition

Pneumonia is defined as an inflammatory reaction in the lower respiratory tract due to infection with an organism that is usually a bacteria, but may be a virus, mycoplasma or rarely a rickettsia, protozoa or fungus.

2 Organisms causing bacterial pneumonia in the community

Before the advent of antibiotics over 95% of lobar pneumonia was due to infection with *Streptococcus pneumoniae*. Although *Streptococcus pneumoniae* is still the most commonly isolated organism, possibly because an antibiotic has been given in many cases before specimens have been collected, at the present time no pathogen is identifiable in a third to one-half of cases of community acquired pneumonia.

Thus depending upon the survey from which the data are taken, at the present time in Britain pneumonia acquired outside hospital is due to *Streptococcus pneumoniae* in about a third to three-quarters of cases, *Haemophilus influenzae* in about 5% of cases, viruses in 5–10% of cases, and other unusual organisms such as *Mycoplasma pneumoniae*, *Legionella pneumophila*, *Staphylococcus aureus*, and other rare organisms in a few cases. Very occasionally tuberculosis may present as pneumonia.

Possibly because studies in the United States have included

more alcoholics, drug addicts and other debilitated patients, in the
United States pneumonia is more frequently due to Gram negative
and staphylococcal infection than in Britain.

3 Symptoms, signs, complications

i   *Symptoms*. The symptoms and signs of pneumonia
encompass a spectrum of varying severity. In the elderly or
debilitated the disease may present with little in the way of
temperature or signs. Usually, however, the patient has prodromal
symptoms of a febrile illness such as malaise, sweating, aches and
pains, and sometimes rigors. There may be a history of a preceding
upper respiratory tract infection. Specific symptoms include
breathlessness, and pleuritic chest pain when the process involves
the pleura. With the exception of legionella or klebsiella
pneumonia, frank haemoptysis is rare and should arouse suspicion
of underlying bronchiectasis or a neoplasm.

ii   *Signs*. The patient may appear flushed and toxic with
tachycardia and tachypnoea. Temperature 39°C or greater and
rigors occur in young people, and are particularly suggestive of
pneumococcal or legionella pneumonia. Cyanosis due to
mismatching of ventilation and perfusion may be seen as a result of
poor aeration of the affected lung.
•   *Within the chest* the signs are variable. Laennec described
the usual sequence of events as crackles followed by bronchial
breathing followed by crackles. Certainly crackles are the
commonest sign, but there may be no abnormal physical signs
despite extensive consolidation on chest x-ray. The classical signs
of consolidation occur in only about a third of patients, and are
dullness to percussion, an increase of tactile and vocal fremitus,
and bronchial breathing that may allow whispering pectoriloquy.
The acoustics of bronchial breathing are explained on page 24. In
addition, a pleural rub may be heard.

iii   *Complications* are pleural effusion, empyema (discussed on
page 302), and abscess formation particularly with staphylococcal,
pneumococcal serotype 3 or Friedländer's pneumonia. Failure of
resolution or recurrent pneumonia should always arouse suspicion
of a lesion obstructing a bronchus, for example a carcinoma or an
inhaled foreign body, or alternatively a systemic disorder such as
diabetes, achalasia or neuromuscular inco-ordination due for
instance to motor neurone disease.

4 Investigations

Many cases of pneumonia are treated in the community without
any investigation. In hospital the following investigations should be
performed:
•   *Total white cell count*. A neutrophilia causing a total white
cell count $> 15 \times 10^9/l$ occurs in about half the cases of
pneumococcal pneumonia, but is less pronounced in pneumonia

of most other causes. In very ill patients the white cell count may be low, and is a poor prognostic sign. In uncomplicated viral pneumonia the white cell count is usually normal.

● *Culture of sputum, blood and any pleural fluid* that can be aspirated should be carried out before antibiotics are given. Sputum culture is positive in about 10% of cases of legionella pneumonia, and up to 50% of cases of pneumococcal pneumonia. In pneumococcal pneumonia blood culture is positive in more than 30% of cases.

● *Gram's stain of the sputum* may be helpful if significant numbers of organisms are seen. However, in practice significant numbers are seen in about only 10-20% of cases of pneumococcal pneumonia.

● *Chest x-ray* confirms the diagnosis, showing either homogeneous shadowing of a lobe, a segment or even a whole lung, or patchy shadowing, particularly at the lung bases. Partial collapse of a lung may be due to mucous plugging, a tumour or aspiration of food, vomitus or a foreign body. Cavitation within the shadowing is rare and suggests staphylococcal, pneumococcal serotype 3 or Friedländer's pneumonia.

● *Serology.* Although only of use retrospectively, a fourfold increase in specific antibody titre in samples taken 10-14 days apart is accepted evidence of infection, and is the usual method of confirming pneumonia due to viruses, *Legionella pneumophila* or *Mycoplasma pneumoniae*.

Pneumonia due to particular organisms and particular situations
Question

5   Write short notes naming the causative organism or organisms and any special clinical or investigative features or particular complications that may arise with the following conditions. What antibiotics are used to treat them?
i   *Pneumonia due to particular organisms:* pneumococcal pneumonia, staphylococcal pneumonia, legionella pneumonia, Friedländer's pneumonia, mycoplasma pneumonia, ornithosis (psittacosis), Q fever, viral pneumonia.
ii   *Pneumonia in special situations:* bacterial pneumonia complicating influenza, pneumonia complicating obstructive airways disease, hospital acquired or nosocomial pneumonia, pneumonia in the immunocompromised patient. What measures may help reduce the likelihood of hospital acquired infection?

Answer

5i   Pneumonia due to particular organisms

● *Pneumococcal pneumonia* is due to *Streptococcus pneumoniae*. A high temperature (39°C or greater) and rigors are suggestive of this type of pneumonia. Classical signs of consolidation occur in about a third of cases. Herpes labialis is a specific feature of the condition and also occurs in about a third of cases. Treatment is along the lines discussed in the answer to question 6.

● *Staphylococcal pneumonia* is due to *Staphylococcus aureus*. Infection may occur as a primary infection at any age, but occurs most commonly as a complication of influenza, or as a result of septicaemia associated with a boil or intravenous drug abuse or as secondary infection of a pulmonary infarct. Cavities may form within the consolidated area, or particularly in cases of septicaemia, multiple thin walled abscesses may form in the lung. Treatment is with flucloxacillin 500 mg 6 hourly. In severe cases the drug should be given with fusidic acid, and initially both should be by intravenous injection.

● *Legionella pneumonia* is due to the Gram negative organism, *Legionella pneumophila*, and is an unusual condition that tends to occur sporadically in small outbreaks. The reservoirs of the organism are humid situations such as the humidifying systems of large buildings, and shower heads. The disease spans a spectrum from a mild respiratory illness to a fatal disease with death from multisystem organ failure. In addition to features such as cough, fever, myalgia and consolidation, in severe cases *the diagnosis is aided by the multisystem nature of the disease* which produces headache, drowsiness and confusion in the nervous system, diarrhoea, vomiting and abdominal pain in the gastrointestinal system, and sometimes renal failure. Haemoptysis occurs in a third of cases. On investigation, although a neutrophilia occurs it is usually not much above $10 \times 10^9/l$, and in about two-thirds of cases is accompanied by lymphopenia $< 1 \times 10^9/l$ and hyponatraemia < 130 mm/l. The diagnosis is confirmed by culture or direct fluorescent antibody staining of organisms in the sputum and lung tissue obtained by biopsy, and retrospectively by serology. Treatment is with erythromycin 500 mg–1 g four times daily for 14 days, initially by intravenous injection in severely ill patients.

● *Friedländer's pneumonia* is due to Friedländer's Gram negative bacillus, *Klebsiella pneumoniae*. It is an uncommon condition with a considerable mortality, and presents with lobar pneumonia that has a tendency to progress to sloughing of the lung, abscess formation and healing by fibrosis. Haemoptysis may occur. Diagnosis is by Gram stain and culture of the sputum. The organism is resistant to the penicillins, but is often sensitive to co-trimoxazole, the cephalosporins, chloramphenicol and gentamicin. Treatment is usually with gentamicin and a cephalosporin for 2–3 days, then when the patient is somewhat better, with gentamicin alone.

● *Mycoplasma pneumonia* is due to *Mycoplasma pneumoniae*, an organism that has features of both a bacterium and a virus. Although it does not have a cell wall it can be grown on culture medium outside living cells, and is sensitive to both erythromycin and tetracycline. Myocoplasma infections have a 3–4 year periodicity throughout the world. Particular prodromal clinical features include headache and malaise. On examination there may be disparity between the paucity of signs in the chest and the extent of consolidation on chest x-ray. There is usually no leucocytosis, but in about 50% of cases the blood contains cold agglutinins which increase several fold in titre over a period of about 2 weeks. Because of the agglutinins, the condition may be complicated by haemolytic anaemia, and also by myocarditis or pleural effusion. Treatment is usually with erythromycin 500 mg four times daily.

●   *Ornithosis (psittacosis)* is due to *Chlamydia psittaci*, an organism that is between a virus and a rickettsia and is found in birds. The illness is caught mainly from parrots, budgerigars, canaries and poultry. The organism may be cultured from sputum and blood. A rising titre of specific antibody may be demonstrated. Treatment is with tetracycline 500 mg four times daily.

●   *Q fever* is due to the rickettsia, *Coxiella burneti*, a small Gram negative bacillus that grows only in cells, and infects animals such as sheep, cows and goats. Infection in humans occurs from inhaling rickettsiae as an aerosol from dried infected tick or animal excretions or from drinking contaminated milk. Headache is a prominent feature of the illness. A granulomatous hepatitis occurs in about a third of patients. Infective endocarditis also occurs occasionally. Treatment is with tetracycline 500 mg three times daily or chloramphenicol 500 mg four times daily.

●   *Primary viral pneumonia* is rare, but may be caused by the influenza virus. Much more commonly pneumonia occurring a few days after the onset of influenza is due to secondary bacterial infection. This is discussed below.

5ii   Pneumonia in special situations

●   *Bacterial pneumonia complicating influenza* occurs as a secondary infection often associated with rapid deterioration and leucopenia a few days after the onset of influenza. The organisms involved are *Haemophilus influenzae*, *Streptococcus pneumoniae* or *Staphylococcus aureus*. Treatment is given intravenously with benzylpenicillin 600–1200 mg (1–2 mega units) 6 hourly, flucloxacillin 500 mg 6 hourly, and ampicillin 500 mg 6 hourly.

●   *Pneumonia complicating chronic obstructive airways disease* is usually due to the organisms associated with exacerbations of the condition, namely *Streptococcus pneumoniae* or *Haemophilus influenzae*, and is treated with a broad spectrum antibiotic such as ampicillin 500 mg four times daily, co-trimoxazole 2 tablets twice daily or trimethoprim 200 mg twice daily.

●   *Hospital acquired or nosocomial pneumonia*. The word nosocomia is derived from Greek and implies disease acquired in hospital. Pneumonia acquired in this situation differs from pneumonia acquired in the community in two important respects. *Firstly it is often due to aspiration; secondly the organisms involved are often unusual*. Patients at particular risk of aspiration and this type of pneumonia are those who are ill in bed, especially if they are suffering from impaired consciousness due to neurological disease or sedative drugs, suppressed immunity, or have undergone a general anaesthetic or abdominal operation. The explanation of the unusual organisms is that the nasopharynx of more than 40% of hospitalised patients is colonised by Gram negative bacilli. As a consequence, *in up to half the cases* of nosocomial pneumonia the infecting organism is a Gram negative bacillus such as *Escherichia coli*, a *Pseudomonas* species, *Klebsiella pneumoniae* or *Bacteroides*. Among the Gram positive organisms, *Staphylococcus aureus* is the commonest, occurring in about 10% of cases. *Streptococcus pneumoniae* causes only about 10% of cases.

Treatment of this type of pneumonia is with a third generation cephalosporin, gentamicin, and if *Bacteroides* is suspected, with metronidazole. Infection with *Staphylococcus aureus* is treated with flucloxacillin.

The risk of nosocomial pneumonia may be reduced by preventing smoking before operation, and by chest physiotherapy and early mobilisation after operation.

● *Pneumonia in the immunosuppressed*. Patients with suppressed immunity due to diseases such as the acquired immune deficiency syndrome (AIDS), reticulosis or leukaemia, or cytotoxic drug therapy are at particular risk of infection. Bacterial pneumonia, tuberculosis or infections with unusual organisms may occur. These include the protozoan, *Pneumocystis carinii*, which may be treated with pentamidine or large doses of co-trimoxazole, viruses such as cytomegalovirus, which may be treated with DHPG and Foscarnet, yeasts such as *Cryptococcus neoformans* and *Candida albicans* and fungi such as *Aspergillus fumigatus*.

Treatment of pneumonia in ordinary clinical practice
Question

6   The previous question dealt with pneumonia due to particular organisms and particular situations. In ordinary clinical practice the infecting organism is usually not known. Detail (i) the general, and (ii) the antibiotic treatment of a moderately ill and a severely ill patient. State the dose and frequency of administration of the drugs.

Answer

6   **Treatment in ordinary clinical practice**

Because the infecting organism is not known in most cases of pneumonia at the time of starting treatment, the answer to this question embraces the management of most cases of pneumonia met with in ordinary clinical practice. The treatment of such a case may be divided into (i) general measures, and (ii) specific antibiotic therapy.

i   *General measures*. Patients with severe pneumonia should be admitted to hospital. Subject to their social conditions, those who are only moderately ill may be treated at home. The patient should be nursed in bed for 2 or 3 days, and encouraged to drink plenty. Maintenance of good hydration aids recovery. Pleuritic chest pain should be treated with aspirin 600 mg or indomethacin 50 mg 3-4 hourly as required. Cyanosis is an indication for continuous oxygen therapy. Very occasionally assisted ventilation is required and may be life saving in those rare cases that develop marked respiratory failure. Physiotherapy is rarely helpful whilst the patient is acutely ill and may be exhausting, but often helps clear secretions during the convalescent phase.

ii   *Antibiotics* are usually given for 7-10 days. Because the organism is usually not known at the onset of the illness, choice of antibiotic is empirical. Usually a broad spectrum agent that is active against both *Streptococcus penumoniae* and *Haemophilus influenzae* such as ampicillin 500 mg is given four times daily. If mycoplasma or legionella pneumonia is suspected erythromycin 500 mg four times per day should be prescribed.

In severely ill patients a regimen that covers all the above pathogens should be given by intravenous bolus injection. The recommended regimen is benzylpenicillin 600-1200 mg (1-2 mega units) 6 hourly and erythromycin 500 mg-1 g 6 hourly for 2-3 days, followed by oral therapy.

Further Reading

Crofton J, Douglas A (1981). *Respiratory Diseases*, 3rd edition. Blackwell Scientific Publications, Oxford. Chapter 9, pneumonia.

Chapter 21
Bronchiectasis, Lung
Abscess and Empyema

Bronchiectasis (i): definition, pathology, causes, Kartagener's syndrome

Questions

1   Define the term 'bronchiectasis'. What are the two main factors leading to the development of bronchiectasis? Which areas of the lungs are usually affected by the condition?

2   Describe the histological changes that occur in the bronchial wall with bronchiectasis.

3   List the main underlying causes of bronchiectasis.

4   Describe Kartagener's syndrome. How may the bronchiectasis associated with it be explained?

Answers

1   Definition

Bronchiectasis is a permanent abnormal dilatation of a bronchus due to damage from prolonged inflammation of the bronchial wall.

The two main factors in the development of bronchiectasis are *obstruction* and *infection* of the bronchi. *Obstruction* may be due to secretions, foreign body or tumour blocking a bronchus, and prevents the normal clearance of secretions by the mucociliary escalator. *Infection* probably damages the bronchial wall by way of the release from trapped neutrophils of tissue damaging enzymes such as elastase.

Because of the effects of gravity upon the mucous secretions, the areas most often affected by bronchiectasis are the lower more dependent parts of the lung, although tumours and foreign bodies may result in localised disease in other parts, and post-primary tuberculosis in disease of the upper lobes.

2   Histological changes

Bronchiectatic saccules are associated with thin fibrotic walls and loss of cartilage. Other changes that occur are hypertrophy of the pseudostratified columnar epithelium, and infiltration of the submucosa with lymphocytes and plasma cells.

3   Underlying main causes of bronchiectasis

●   *Childhood measles and whooping cough* due to infected secretions obstructing the bronchi.

●   *Tuberculosis*. Extensive *post-primary tuberculosis* in the upper lobes may lead to bronchiectasis of the upper lobes that drains by gravity. *Primary tuberculosis* may result in bronchiectasis of the right middle lobe due to obstruction of the bronchus by compression from enlarged adjacent hilar lymph nodes.

- *Foreign body* obstructing a bronchus.
- *Carcinoma* obstructing a bronchus.
- *Aspergillosis. Proximal* bronchiectasis may occur due to inflammation and plugging of bronchi in asthmatics who develop bronchopulmonary aspergillosis.
- *Cystic fibrosis:* due to infected secretions obstructing a bronchus.
- *Hypogammaglobulinaemia:* due to infected secretions obstructing the bronchi.
- *Kartagener's syndrome*—discussed below.

4   Kartagener's syndrome

This is the association of sinusitis, bronchiectasis, situs inversus (dextrocardia and transposition of the abdominal viscera) and infertility. The explanation of the bronchiectasis, sinusitis and infertility associated with the condition is that the respiratory cilia and the tail of the sperm share a common motor system. In Kartagener's syndrome this system is defective, producing immobile sperms and immobile cilia.

Bronchiectasis (ii): clinical features, investigation, treatment
Questions

5   What are (i) the symptoms, and (ii) the signs of bronchiectasis?

6   What are the complications of bronchiectasis?

7   What changes may be seen on chest x-ray in cases of bronchiectasis? What is bronchography? What are the indications for performing it?

8   Describe the treatment of bronchiectasis. What are the indications for surgery?

Answers

5   Symptoms and signs

i   The *symptoms* span a wide spectrum that is related to the cause and extent of the disease. Bronchiectasis involving only a segment of a lobe may be asymptomatic or productive of purulent sputum only after a cold. At the other end of the spectrum, patients with extensive disease may produce more than a cupful of purulent sputum daily, and may be breathless, and experience recurrent haemoptysis, pleurisy and episodes of fever and pneumonia.

ii   The *signs* vary with the extent of the disease. There may be no signs, although more typically late crackles are audible over the affected area. The breath may be foul smelling. Clubbing of fingers may be present.

6 Complications

These include haemoptysis, chronic airways obstruction that is often amenable to bronchodilators, recurrent pneumonia, lung abscess, empyema, cor pulmonale and respiratory failure, and amyloidosis.

7 Chest x-ray changes; bronchography

Chest x-ray may be normal, but in most cases increased markings are visible over the affected areas due to patchy consolidation, collapse and crowding of bronchi. Dilated bronchi may be visible in the form of tubes and ring shadows that may contain fluid levels. *Bronchography* involves the introduction of radio-opaque contrast medium into the bronchial tree, and is performed mainly in cases in which surgery is contemplated:
a   to obtain a definite diagnosis, and
b   to assess the extent of the disease.

8 Treatment

Smoking should be discouraged. Patients with mild disease require no more than a course of a broad spectrum antibiotic such as ampicillin, co-trimoxazole or tetracycline during active chest infections signalled by fever and increased production of purulent sputum. A few patients with severe disease respond only to large doses of antibiotics, for instance amoxycillin 3 g twice daily for 10 days. Patients producing large amounts of sputum should be instructed to do regular postural drainage for about 10 minutes on rising and before retiring, and if necessary during the day. This involves lying head down on a sloping bed or board or over a chair in such a position as to drain the bronchiectatic area by gravity and coughing, and if necessary by percussion of the chest. *Surgery* is reserved for those few patients with chronic severe symptoms not responding to medical treatment who have bronchographically demonstrated local disease. Surgery is contraindicated by widespread disease or chronic airways obstruction.

Lung abscess: definition, causes, clinical features
Questions

9   Define the term 'lung abscess'.
10   List the causes of lung abscess.
11i   To which sites in the lungs is aspiration likely to occur?
  ii   What organisms are likely in lung abscess due to aspiration?
12   Discuss the symptoms, signs and investigation of suspected lung abscess.
13   How is lung abscess treated?

Answers

9   Definition

Lung abscess is an infective lesion within the lung that leads to suppuration and necrosis of lung tissue usually with formation of a cavity.

10   Causes

● *Aspiration of infected secretions or vomitus.* This is particularly likely in patients whose cough reflex is suppressed due to unconsciousness from head injury, stroke, epilepsy, anaesthesia, alcohol or drugs. Aspiration may also occur in patients with achalasia and neuromuscular inco-ordination.
● *Obstruction of a bronchus* due to a carcinoma or foreign body such as an aspirated tooth.
● *Infection of a pulmonary infarct.*
● *Pneumonia,* particularly staphylococcal or Friedländer's.
● *Spread from a subphrenic or hepatic abscess,* particularly from an amoebic abscess, actinomycosis or hydatid cyst.

11   Aspiration in the lung; associated organisms

i   The site in the lung to which aspiration is likely to occur is determined by the anatomy of the lung and the effect of the patient's position upon the gravitational drainage of the lung.
● *In the supine position* aspiration occurs into the apical segment of the lower lobe or the posterior segment of the upper lobe.
● *In the upright position* aspiration occurs into the right lower lobe.
● *In the lateral position* aspiration occurs into the axillary parts of the anterior and posterior segments of the upper lobe.

ii   *Organisms associated with aspiration.* Lung abscess resulting from aspiration contains the mixture of organisms found in the nasopharynx. Even in health the secretions of the oral pharynx contain about 10^8 anaerobes/ml such as fusiforms, *Bacteroides* species and anaerobic cocci. To this Gram negative bacilli and *Staphylococcus aureus* are added in hospital patients.

12   Symptoms, signs and investigations

Lung abscess presents like pneumonia with pyrexia, malaise, cough, shivers and sometimes pleuritic chest pain. After about a week the abscess discharges into a bronchus and the patient coughs up a large amount of pus and blood stained material. Unless the abscess is near the surface, there may be a few signs in the chest.
● Chest x-ray early in the illness shows the affected area to be opaque. When the abscess has discharged a cavity, often containing a fluid level, may be seen. Blood and sputum should be cultured

before antibiotics are given. Bronchoscopy should be performed

a   to collect secretions for culture from the appropriate area without contamination by the upper airways, and

b   to see if a carcinoma or foreign body is present.

13 Treatment

The anaerobes involved in lung abscess due to aspiration usually respond to benzylpenicillin given by intravenous bolus 1200–1800 mg (2–3 mega units) four times daily until the patient improves at which stage treatment may be changed to phenoxymethylpenicillin 1 gram orally four times daily until healing has occurred. Metronidazole should be added if there are doubts about the sensitivity of the organisms. Infection due to staphylococci should be treated with flucloxacillin, and due to *Klebsiella* with a cephalosporin and gentamicin. Postural drainage with percussion aids the clearance of pus.

With this treatment resolution occurs in 70–80% of lung abscesses. Failure of resolution should re-arouse suspicion of an underlying carcinoma, and is an indication for surgical excision.

Empyema: definition, causes, clinical features

Questions

14   Define the term 'empyema'. What are its causes?

15   What are the symptoms and signs of empyema?

16   How is the condition diagnosed and treated?

Answers

14 Definition and causes

Empyema is the occurrence of infected fluid or frank pus in the pleural cavity.

It may occur as part of a pneumonia (often pneumococcal), or through spread of infection into the pleural space from a lung abscess, subphrenic abscess, infection of the mediastinum or penetrating chest wound.

15 Symptoms and signs

Typically empyema occurs a few days after the onset of pneumococcal pneumonia and is accompanied by a recurrence of fever, anorexia, feeling unwell, sweats, malaise and sometimes pleuritic chest pain. Examination of the chest reveals signs of pleural effusion. Chronic empyema causes chronic unwellness, weight loss, sometimes a low grade fever, clubbing of the fingers and a normochromic anaemia.

16 Diagnosis and treatment

The presence of fluid within the chest is confirmed by chest x-ray. A definitive diagnosis is made by needle aspiration of turbid fluid or frank pus which should be cultured both aerobically and anaerobically, and if necessary examined by Ziehl-Neelsen stain and cultured for tuberculosis.

The principles of the treatment of empyema are obliteration of the pleural space and eradication of infection. Thin fluid may be treated by daily aspiration or indwelling drain and the systemic administration of an appropriate antibiotic chosen as a result of sensitivity testing of the organism. With thick pus surgical clearance of the pleural space and decortication of the lung are usually required.

Further Reading

Crofton J, Douglas A (1981) *Respiratory Diseases*, 3rd edition. Blackwell Scientific Publications, Oxford. Chapters 10, empyema; 11, lung abscess; 24, bronchiectasis.

Weatherall DJ, Ledingham JGG, Warrell DA (eds) (1987). *Oxford Textbook of Medicine*, 2nd edition. Oxford University Press, Oxford. The suppurative lung diseases, pp 15.100-6.

Index